Comments  first edition of

The Ostomy Book

"Wow!. . . All I could ask now is that everyone could read the book."

Donald P. Binder
Former Executive Director
United Ostomy Association

"The Ostomy Book combines in a most favorable way, factual information with sensitivity. . .For anyone about to undergo ostomy surgery or in the immediate post-operative period and for their families, this book should be compulsory reading. . .For those with professional involvement in the care of ostomates, the book will have equal appeal. . . .I recommend it unreservedly..."

J. R. Kirkpatrick, MD
Professor of Surgery
Member, Professional Advisory Boards
United Ostomy Association
International Ostomy Association

THE OSTOMY BOOK

BARBARA DORR MULLEN

KERRY ANNE McGINN, RN, BSN, MA, OCN

THE OSTOMY
BOOK ❋ *Living*
Comfortably with Colostomies,
Ileostomies, and Urostomies

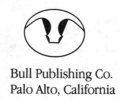

Bull Publishing Co.
Palo Alto, California

Copyright 1980, 1992 Barbara Dorr Mullen and Kerry Anne McGinn

Bull Publishing Company
P.O. Box 208
Palo Alto CA 94302-0208
(415) 322-2855

ISBN 0-923521-12-7

Distributed in the U.S. by:
Publishers Group West
4065 Hollis Street
Emeryville, CA 94608

Library of Congress Cataloging-in-Publication Data

Mullen, Barbara Dorr.

The ostomy book : living comfortably with colostomies, ileos-tomies, and urostomies / by Barbara Dorr Mullen, Kerry Anne McGinn.
  p. cm.
  Includes index.

ISBN 0-923521-12-7

1. Ostomates—Care. 2. Ostomates—Rehabilitation. I. McGinn, Kerry Anne. II. Title.

[DNLM: 1. Colostomy—popular works. 2. Ileostomy—popular works. 3. Urinary Diversion—popular works. WI 520 M958o]
RD540M97 1992
617.5'54—dc20
DNLM/DLC
for Library of Congress   91-36233
                                                          CIP

Cover Design: Paula Schlosser Design
Production Manager: Helen O'Donnell
Illustrators: Susan Klug, Ken Miller, Lois Stanfield
Compositor: Typola
Text Face: Garamond
Printer: Bookcrafters, Inc.

Dedicated, with affection,

to everyone who has an ostomy—and

to all those who care for them.

Contents

	Dear Reader	vii
Chapter 1	I'm Going to Have a What?	1
Chapter 2	What is an Ostomy?	13
Chapter 3	It's Your Body	26
Chapter 4	Before Surgery	33
Chapter 5	Surgery, and Just After	43
Chapter 6	On the Mend	50
Chapter 7	But How Do You Really Feel?	60
Chapter 8	That Strange Big World Out There	67
Chapter 9	Permanent Colostomies: Changes and Choices	73
Chapter 10	Ileostomies and Alternatives	86
Chapter 11	Life Without A Built-in Bladder	101
Chapter 12	Pouches and the Skin They Touch	114
Chapter 13	Pouch Skills	132
Chapter 14	Temporary Ostomies	144
Chapter 15	Eating Well	162
Chapter 16	Catnaps, Strolls, and Good Belly Laughs	172
Chapter 17	You're Looking Great!	180
Chapter 18	What About Sex?	186
Chapter 19	A Touch of Pregnancy	198
Chapter 20	Children with Ostomies	205
Chapter 21	A Word to the Teenagers	213
Chapter 22	Check-ups and Follow-ups	220
Chapter 23	Work? Of Course!	231
Chapter 24	Swimming, Skiing and Other Diversions	241
Chapter 25	The Other Side of the World	250
Chapter 26	Enterostomal Therapy: A New Profession	261
Chapter 27	The Phoenix: UOA and Its Ancestors	273
Chapter 28	In the Family	285
	Addresses To Know	289
	Glossary	291
	Index	310

List of Illustrations

Digestive and Urinary Tracts   16
Sigmoid Colostomy   17
Ileostomy   17
Urostomy (Ileal Conduit)   18
Constructing a Stoma   23
Sigmoid Colostomy   77
Irrigating a Colostomy   82–85
Ileostomy   92
Continent Ileostomy with Catheter   93
Ileoanal Reservoir   95
Urostomy (Illeal Conduit)   105
Night Drainage System   110
Urostomy Pouches   117
Drainable Pouch   117
Security Pouch for Colostomy   118
Pouches   124
Convexity   127
Changing a Pouch   133–142
Loop Ostomy   149
Construction of a Loop Ostomy   151
Double-Barrel Ostomy   152
End Ostomy and Hartmann's Pouch   153
Pouching a Double-Barrel Ostomy   156
Pouching a Loop Ostomy   157

Dear Reader,

This book happened because Barbara, a free-lance writer, had a colostomy. And was curious. Why didn't anyone talk about ostomy surgery?

Barbara's daughter Kerry, an RN and an experienced writer, joined the project later.

For two reasons, we belive The Ostomy Book is a rather special book.

First, so far as we know, it's the first book for the general reader on ostomy surgery, a group of abdominal operations which save thousands of lives every year, yet remain wrapped in secrecy, taboos, and nonsense. It's time the windows were open.

Second, it's a book that's had such an enthusiastic group of helpers, lay and professional, that it's almost embarrassing to put only our names on the cover as authors.

After joining the United Ostomy Association, Barbara sent a plea for help to the central office. The results were beautiful and overwhelming. Ostomates from all over— Nova Scotia, New York, Chicago, Medicine Hat, Texas, California, the Oregon coast and elsewhere responded with letters, personal accounts and newsletters. The message was clear—we need the book. One of our favorites came from Muriel Bastin in Monterey, California, who told us that she's well enough following her ostomy surgery to drive her pink Buick again and says she's just gotten her driver's license renewed—at age 94!

We are grateful to David Bull, our enthusiastic and supportive publisher; Susan Klug, our talented illustrator; and Gloria Fisher, our dedicated typist.

The following people carefully reviewed the manuscript and enriched it with their wisdom and information: Victor Alterescu, RN, ET; Donald Binder, Executive Director of the United Ostomy Association; Gerry Cameron, RN, ET; Catharine Flinn; Katherine F. Jeter, EdD, ET; James R. Kirkpatrick, MD; Edith Lenneberg, ET; Lotte Moise; Karen Moise, RN; Carol Norris, PhD; Robert Reinker, MD; George Schreiber, MD; Valerie Stoller, RN; and Michael Wise, MD.

We also thank the many persons whose stories appear in this book (and the Ostomy Quarterly for permission to reprint several of them), and the many people who shared their experiences with us in letter and conversation. Without them, this book never would have come to be.

And finally, we are grateful to Kerry's husband, Art, and their children—Michael, Kathleen, John, and Steven—for unbelievable patience with the book.

Fondly,

Barbara Dorr Mullen
Kerry Anne McGinn
April, 1980

Dear Reader,

Almost twelve years have passed since the first copy of The Ostomy Book appeared. In those years, much has happened, both in the ostomy world and in our own lives. In the ostomy world, new equipment, surgical procedures, and resources have appeared. Statistics and treatments have changed and so have the things that the person with an ostomy should know. (It's obviously time to update a book when every single one of the addresses is outdated!)

In our own lives: My mother, Barbara Dorr Mullen, died—very peacefully with family and friends around her. She was elated that The Ostomy Book was becoming a treasured friend to so many people. Her spirit still hovers...

What has been updated in this revision is the information. The personal stories (including my mother's) remain unchanged, or largely so. This means a little "time warp" on occasion, since the experiences, initials after people's names, and such are several years old.

Again, there are so many people to thank, especially publisher David Bull (enthusiastic and supportive, as always), Helen O'Donnell of Bull Publishing (who makes it all come together), and Ken Miller who drew the new illustrations for the revised edition.

I am grateful to the people who reviewed the manuscript and added to its accuracy and clarity: Karen Alterescu, RN, MS, ET, nurse coordinator of the Inflammatory Bowel Disease Center of California Pacific Medical Center (CPMC), San Francisco; Linda King Aukett, board member of the United Ostomy Association; Jeanne Colberg, RN, ET, editor of the "Ostomy World" column in the Ostomy Quarterly; and James W. Fleshman, MD, colorectal surgeon, Jewish Hospital at Washington University Medical Center, St. Louis, Missouri.

And a big thank you to the people who graciously

allowed me to interview them or who helped update individual chapters: *Karen Alterescu, RN, MS, ET; Susan Barbour, RN, MS, ET, University of California Medical Center, San Francisco; J. Michael Berry, MD, medical oncologist, CPMC; Joseph Ignatius, MD, general surgeon, CPMC, and editor of The Surgical Index; Valerie Marron, RN, CETN, Kaiser-Permanente Medical Center, San Francisco; Marilyn Mau, former president, United Ostomy Association; Melinda Parker, RD, MS, dietitian, CPMC; Thomas Russell, MD, colorectal surgeon, CPMC; Joseph Spaulding, MD, urologic surgeon, CPMC; and James Stricker, MD, colorectal surgeon, Kaiser-Permanente Medical Center, San Francisco. Thank you also to Thomas Buch, April Gimlen and Cy Smith of UOA.*

My thanks to all of you! You made the project possible.

And, of course, I will always be grateful to my husband Art, my children Michael, Kathleen, John (and wife Susan) and Steven (and wife Cathy), and my father, Robert Mullen.

Fondly,

Kerry Anne McGinn
December 1991

CHAPTER 1 ❋ *I'm Going to Have a What?*

A human body is an ingenious
assembly of portable plumbing.
Christopher Morley

As my friend Tom says, you never realize how many yellow cars there are—until you buy a yellow car.

Until July, 1976, I had no idea that hundreds of thousands of Americans had gained longer lives, thanks to a surgical change I'd barely heard of—an *ostomy*. Nor did I guess that I'd be one of the lucky ones who would receive such a bonus of time.

Nor that I would need it. . .

Though the apple trees and primroses probably bloomed on schedule that spring, I'd been too busy focusing on black clouds and mud puddles to notice them. My work wasn't going well, my body seemed to have lost its bounce, and I'd been in a rut so long I felt bruised. If I could swing it, maybe a vacation—a week or two on Puget Sound—would help? What I needed was a change.

What I got were changes. Instead of two weeks moseying up the coast to the Sound, I got four weeks and two days in a pink hospital room in San Francisco with a distant view of Golden Gate Park. Instead of fresh salmon and wild blackberry pie, there were bland, hot cereal and jello on blue plastic trays.

Those changes were temporary. I also got a slight change in my plumbing—*a colostomy*—and that's permanent, but less trouble than I expected, and cause for rejoicing. No matter what I used to think!

It all started on a Wednesday in July, near the end of a long-postponed physical. That had gone well. The doctor, Michael Wise, and I were pleased at my rich blood, marvelous blood pressure, all kinds of good signs.

Until that undignified last lap. My body was bent like a tent on the examining table so Dr. Wise could look into my rectum through a special tube called a *sigmoidoscope*. He'd been talking to put me at ease. Then he stopped. After our banter, the silence was scary.

"There," he said, after a few moments. "Just relax a minute, Barb, while I get someone else to look at this." Someone else was a doctor who specialized in problems of the digestive tract. He agreed the small odd growth looked suspicious. They'd better do a biopsy; they snipped out a tiny sample of the suspicious tissue so that it could be examined under a microscope to see what was causing the changes.

When my daughter Kerry and I returned Friday morning for the results, a cup of coffee (a welcome if ominous courtesy) was waiting for me. Dr. Wise didn't mince words. The sample tissue appeared to be maverick: a young cancer. "So—we want you to come back early Monday morning, ready to stay a week or two. We'll do a few more tests and then, probably, surgery."

"What kind of surgery?"

"A colostomy."

A colostomy! I didn't like the sound of that, though I wasn't really sure what it was. Besides, this whole business was absurd! My digestion had always been excellent.

Other people got intestinal flu or worried about irregularity; I hadn't even taken a laxative since I was ten years old.

Yet, if I'm honest, it wasn't a total surprise. There'd been small omens, all that spring. In March, suspecting an ulcer, I'd made a note in my journal: "Some concern about bleeding from the bowel. Try to avoid *all* raw and rough foods and see if it goes away." Later in the month, I added a happy P.S. to myself: "Gone away. Probably just minor."

Even such brief interest in my bowels embarrassed me, I remember. I'd had the usual childhood indoctrination in things we don't talk about. Later, reading Freud had persuaded me that concern with elimination was a dangerous symptom of regression to a childish stage and not (as I know now) intelligent attention due the only body I've got. But, though I tried to ignore them, there were small continuing problems in April, May and June. Not much blood but some.

Of course I knew a change in bowel habits is one of the seven danger signals the American and Canadian Cancer Societies warn us about, but that couldn't mean me. I had enough trouble without worrying about that. . .

"Any questions?" Dr. Wise brought me back to July.

"No." I had a million but couldn't find the words.

All that weekend, melodrama, numbness, and a small trace of common sense fought it out. I didn't know much about hospitals, and remember wondering silly things. Could I develop film there? Take my typewriter? I tried to stuff Saturday and Sunday so full of friends and chores I couldn't think about Monday, or touch my fears. Still, I wrote a few frightened farewell letters to old friends. "I'll be OK," I sniffled, "probably. . .although the doctor does suspect cancer. . . ."

When I checked into the hospital Monday I felt fine, though unreal—the stand-in for a documentary film, starring someone else. Further tests would show how wrong they were, and I'd go home. But more tests all said the same thing: rectal cancer, young but growing and dangerous.

I still didn't believe it.

Surgery would be the next Monday. Besides frequent visits from my daughter and her family, three other things cheered me during that week of waiting.

Recently, I'd finally read *All Creatures Great and Small.* Inspired by veterinarian James Herriot's account, I found myself identifying with the animals he'd treated. As doctor after doctor examined me, remembering that book helped. I was less a person brought low by a vast dose of bubblegum-flavored castor oil than an ailing cow with the scours.

The day we'd gotten the diagnosis, Kerry (with some faint memory of an organization for people with this peculiar surgery) looked in the phone book under "Colostomy," called, and learned that the Golden Gate Chapter of the *United Ostomy Association* met that very night in San Francisco.

Though I didn't go with her, that meeting cheered us both. "They're an amazing group," she reported, "men and women of all ages, great fun, and most of them seemed to feel great." Kerry had won two prizes at the meeting: a new dish towel and a bottle of champagne. Good omens. Not so much winning as discovering that people who had ostomies were lively enough to think of things like prizes.

One of the women had convulsed them with a story from her trip to Hawaii.

"You mean people with ostomies travel that far?"

"You know they do. And anyway, that's not the point. This woman had always wanted to go to a nude beach, even before her surgery, but she'd never had the nerve. In Hawaii, she decided to risk it, with just a camera over her shoulder and a daisy-sprigged ostomy pouch on her belly. She'd worried about what people would say, but nobody paid any attention, except for one person who said, 'What a neat way to carry your film!' "

That silly happy story heartened us all week, and there was hope as well as information in the brochures Kerry had picked up at the UOA meeting. I read them until they were limp—stained with coffee, and probably a few tears.

Basically, I learned, there are three common types of abdominal ostomies. All are surgically-constructed detours in which a channel of elimination is rerouted, so waste (feces or urine) is expelled through a small new exit, the *stoma*, in the abdominal wall.

In a colostomy—the commonest and the kind they said I would have—part of the colon is removed or disconnected; the rectum and anus may be removed. The end of the remaining colon is brought to the surface through the skin of the abdomen and stitched in place. Cancer of the colon or rectum is one of our most common internal cancers and is the most frequent reason for a permanent colostomy; there are all sorts of reasons for temporary colostomies. Colostomy surgery, the UOA brochure promised, saves lives or makes them longer than they would be without surgery. Now that I've met some people who've had their colostomies for twenty or thirty years, I believe it.

An *ileostomy* is sometimes necessary for severe *ulcerative colitis* or *Crohn's disease*. In this case, the entire colon is removed or disconnected, and all or part of the rectum may be removed. The end of the remaining ileum, the last part of the small intestine, is brought through the skin of the abdomen, folded like the neck of a turtleneck sweater, and stitched in place as a stoma. The result, like a miracle, is often an instant cure.

The third type of ostomy is a *urostomy*, or *urinary diversion*. In this operation, the bladder is removed or bypassed and urine is redirected through the opening in the skin to a leakproof, external *pouch* (sometimes called an *appliance*, or even a bag). This surgery can be done to extend life or cure disease. Sometimes it is performed to end months or years of dribbling of urine.

Before surgery, I was less interested in all these anatomical details than in hearing about the lives people led after such surgery. Thanks to one sad true story I knew, I imagined I might be bedridden or at least housebound for a long time. This, I learned, was unlikely unless I was silly enough to choose to hide. People who'd had ostomies were skating, skiing, dancing, making love, and having babies. They swam, jogged, managed large corporations, preached, piloted airplanes, even rode Brahma bulls in rodeos!

And there were so many of them. Of *us*, I amended, somewhat tentatively. I'd thought such far-out, oddball surgery must be rare—I'd not heard much about it—but ostomies are relatively common. Some estimate the annual total at more than 70,000 ostomy operations in the United States and Canada alone, some temporary and some permanent, changes happening to people of all ages, from newborn babies with birth defects to great-grandparents with bowel obstructions.

Book learning is all very well, but right then I needed comfort and reassurance more than facts. My next piece of luck was remembering my friend Irv. Though I'd never asked for details, I'd heard whispers about some mysterious but life-saving rearrangement of his intestines. An ostomy! Since Irv and a friend of his had stayed with me while they were on a bicycle trip that spring, I knew he was in grand health now, whatever they'd done to him.

Irv came to visit, as soon as he got my message.

"It's no big deal, Barb. Only another kind of challenge, and you like challenges."

"Some kinds. I like to pick them."

"Sometimes the unexpected ones are better."

"I hope you're right."

Prickly though I was, Irv's visit proved a comfort. So did other visitors, cards and calls and books and flowers. Reassuring, but still unreal. Why did *I* need get-well cards!

The surgeon, Robert Reinker, allowed plenty of time for us to talk the day before surgery, and was sympathetic as he showed me what they planned to do and where, drawing on my belly with a wide brown felt-tip pen.

"You'll put the darned thing low enough so I can still wear a bikini, won't you!"

"No promises but I'll try, Barb, and there are sexy one-piece bathing suits, you know."

Surgery was just like the TV doctor dramas had taught me: blood transfusions, a tangle of tubes, many hours in the recovery room with nurses hovering. And enough drowse so it was still hard to believe they'd done anything at all—until I looked.

It took me several days to find the courage to do that. Under a bandage, a long and primitive-looking incision straggled up the middle of my abdomen. With those big black stitches, not even neat, I looked like a badly trussed turkey (though you usually use white string for that). I cried when I saw how they'd slashed through my once neat navel.

Slightly east of the incision, a small, clear plastic bag was adhered to my abdomen over the new opening, the stoma. Although this *thing* was both symbol and means for my new way of elimination, I found it harder to accept than the incision. It was so red! Maybe, as it healed, it would fade? No, a stoma gets smaller with time but the color remains poster bright, the natural color of the intestine of which it's still a part.

Behind me, where my anus had been, I felt rather than saw another loosely-basted incision, well buttressed with drainage pads. It hurt.

Looking at what they'd done finally made the changes

almost real, and brought the first wave of sorrow out into the open. Sorrow and sometimes anger, splattering out in brief flurries over trifles. Why did this happen to me? I'd always eaten my spinach.

The tears embarrassed me, and so did the black moods, but I learned grieving only *seems* irrational and childish— it's a necessary step in accepting a loss. Until things healed a little, my body image was askew and my post-operative depression normal, even healthy.

In that drowsy post-surgical time, filled with assorted discomforts but little real pain, everyone pestered me to do a great many things I had little (though increasing) interest in doing. Walk up and down the long halls. Stretch. Breathe deeply. Finish your chicken broth. Smile. Swallow this. Swallow that. Turn over. Learn to take care of your stoma. I loved them all, or most of them, if only they'd leave me alone. . .

But learning to manage my stoma couldn't be postponed forever. With an ostomy, we lose the muscular control we've depended on ever since we were first toilet trained. Regulating the bowels or urine flow in one way or another is essential—physically, psychologically, and socially.

Though I'd read about the choices people with colostomies have, I balked at trying them. Dr. Reinker said he'd have an *ET* come to see me. From my cram reading I knew an ET is an *enterostomal therapist*, a professional who is expert at helping people learn to cope with all kinds of ostomies, assisting with both technical know-how and the psychological adjustment to being different from what we used to be. (Now, almost all ETs are registered nurses as well: *ET nurses.*) But why did I need an expert to teach me how to go to the bathroom?

Jean Alvers, ET, came that evening after dinner. The day had been one long sniffle, and I was stretched out, awash with melancholy, when she bounced in, smiling so warmly I thought she was ten feet tall! (Weeks later, I realized she's shorter than I am.) Jean has an ostomy, too; later I learned that she was one of the pioneers who'd helped develop the profession of enterostomal therapy, many years before. Now, there are close to 2,500 ET nurses in the United States and Canada. Real training centers have replaced early ingenuity.

With the help of Jean's spunk and know-how, I began to see an ostomy was not without hope, and even humor. And to believe problems could be solved, one at a time. The next morning when a nurse announced she was going to do such and such, I shook my head. "I'm going to do it; you may watch if you wish."

With help from what seemed like hundreds of people, I'd begun to reclaim my own body *and* my own autonomy. I'd stopped being the colostomy in the corner bed. I began again to be Barbara who had had colostomy surgery—along with measles, chicken pox, flea bites, sunburn, diphtheria, whooping cough, hepatitis, and assorted other maladies from which I'd also recovered. Strong though fuzzy convictions about my responsibility for my own body revived as I asked more questions, and balked some, knowing I had to be a working member of my treatment team.

I began walking farther each day, not because Dr. Reinker or a nurse said I must, but because I said so. The weekend before I was discharged, I dressed, picked up my two-hour pass, and went for a long walk, halfway round the lake in a nearby park. On my way, I stopped to marvel at every dandelion, every wind-bent tree, every ugly mutt chasing gulls. Part of getting well seemed to be rediscovering how wonderful life was, in spite of everything. Or because! The changes I'd had—and the risks taken—brought life into new focus. I began to sense what people meant when they said surgery could be a time of growth as well as pain, pain that was becoming harder and harder to remember, or even imagine.

Leaving the hospital was a bigger wrench than I'd expected, in spite of 5 a.m. blood pressure readings and other nuisances, and there were shaky patches in the weeks and months ahead. Unscheduled naps. Shaky legs. Storms of tears, blowing up out of nowhere. I didn't enjoy my first swim, or my second—but the third was great.

As for the *thing* part, soon I forgot all about it for hours at a time. Once in a while, I still look at it with surprise and even rare dismay, but it's far less trouble than I imagined and a small price to pay for life.

Though I'd worried some, friends surprised me. A few seemed embarrassed; most were supportive. Some asked about my revised plumbing with cheerful vulgarity. I found such plain speaking more helpful than shy whispers.

Judy asked so many questions as we soaked up sun on her deck one balmy afternoon, I finally asked if she wanted to see it.

"Yes," she said, dubious but determined.

When she'd looked, she seemed disappointed. "Is that all?"

Yup, that's it. The mark is a small one and, for most of us, the inconvenience is minor. That's just one of the things I've learned talking to many new friends, a number of whom just happen to have ostomies as well as being horse breeders, joggers, writers of historical romances, commercial artists, teachers, water skiers, undertakers, backpackers, and much else.

When I was ready, I took a trip, only instead of heading north to Puget Sound as I'd planned before surgery, I went south to San Diego where the United Ostomy Association's annual conference was being held that year. Almost 1500 of us from all over the United States and Canada, and from farther away—Sweden, England, Germany, India and Japan—gathered to compare notes and learn. And to rejoice because of the good things that had happened to us, thanks to slight changes in our plumbing.

Unhappily, not all ostomy surgeries have such satisfactory endings. More would, *if* they were done sooner. To ensure that, we'll have to become more willing to listen when our bodies try to tell us something, instead of turning a deaf ear, as I tried to do.

And we'll have to get better at plain speaking. Openness about ostomies is still a critical problem. Celebrities and the media have been willing to talk about a mastectomy, a vasectomy or almost anything else, but are not so ready to talk about an ostomy. The media features vampires, every variety of sexual pleasure and problem, all kinds of diseases—you name it. Everything but ostomies.

It's silly, if you think about it. The upper end of the digestive tract is loaded with status, prestige—and profit. The success of gourmet restaurants, cookbook writers, fast and slow food chains, makers of lipstick and toothpaste attest to that.

The lower end is also loaded with profit. Laxatives, diarrhea remedies, hemorrhoid salves, toilet bowl cleaners, all are sold in our living rooms, via the euphemisms of TV. But, the minute food leaves the stomach and begins its life-building journey through the digestive canal, it's reclassified as hush-hush, the butt of third-grade jokes and four-letter words, no longer a subject for honest, open conversation.

I write about what happened to me because I believe secrecy about ostomy surgery can be as malignant as cancer; lives are lost in that kind of dark. Too many people with ostomies, shocked by the sudden changes in their bodies, don't know how much help is available. As long as press, radio, and TV are largely silent, how can they find out there are trained professionals *and* trained volunteers, ready to help? Or clinics where problems can be solved? Easy-to-use pouches to contain body wastes, and conferences to lift their spirits?

Some don't learn soon enough that an ostomy is a chance worth taking. Victims of whispers, they postpone or refuse surgery which could have been life-saving, because of their own fears or (worse) those of their doctors, families, friends.

As Irv told me, that night in the hospital, an ostomy is only another kind of challenge. There aren't many limits on what we do, where we go, or the kind of fun we choose, unless we impose them ourselves.

I'm grateful for all my luck—early diagnosis, skilled surgery, good aftercare, and bushels of encouragement.

And delighted to report that this was a great spring for apple blossoms and primroses. They bloomed their heads off and, this time, I was watching.

CHAPTER 2 *What is an Ostomy?*

They say there's a well-preserved Egyptian mummy with what looks like an abdominal ostomy. Unfortunately, the physician left no record of why, or how, nor any clue about how it was managed. . .

An *ostomy* is a surgically-made *opening into* the body. The kind of ostomy we're interested in is the passageway a surgeon constructs through the abdominal wall as an exit for body waste, either feces or urine. Such a change becomes necessary when the normal channel of elimination cannot be used because of illness, accident or birth defect. A new outlet must be developed.

Ostomy refers to the total change the surgeon makes. *Ostomate* is one common term for a person who undergoes this change in personal plumbing (or *ostomist* in some countries). The new opening one can see on the abdomen is called a *stoma*.

There are three general categories of these abdominal outlet ostomies. A *colostomy* is the rerouting of the colon (large intestine). This change may be permanent or temporary. *Ileostomy* describes such a detour in the ileum, the last section of the small intestine. *Urostomy* covers a number of surgical procedures that redirect urine to the outside of the body when the bladder or another part of the urinary tract must be bypassed or removed. Another name for any of these ostomies is *enterostomy*, or opening into the digestive tract; that's the term, taken from two ancient Greek words, that gives enterostomal therapy nurses their name.

Close to a million people in North America, ranging from infants to great grandparents, know what an ostomy really means—because they have one. Among them may be:

JOE, a newly retired engineer. During a check-up before a world cruise, he's shocked when his doctor discovers rectal cancer and schedules the surgery which will result in a colostomy. He's never heard of such a thing. It doesn't soothe Joe when his doctor points out that cancer involving the colon or rectum remains one of our commonest cancers. (Doctors discover nearly 150,000 cases every year, with about one-third in the rectum, two-thirds in the colon. Often it's a slow-growing cancer, and most of the deaths could be prevented with early diagnosis and treatment.) What about Joe's cruise?

SUSAN, a beautiful and energetic toddler. The doctor explains that Susan's urine is not moving out of the body as it should, but is backing up to injure her kidneys. Other means to solve the problem haven't worked, so now Susan's doctor recommends a urostomy. Susan's parents are horrified. Will Susan ever be able to lead a normal life? What will other children say?

MARCIE, a freshman in college. She's so miserable with severe inflammatory bowel disease that her once-active social and academic life is now a memory, growing fainter each day. Now her doctor recommends surgery to remove the unhealthy part of her digestive tract. Her surgeon plans to construct a new internal reservoir where her rectum is now, but tells Marcie that she will need a temporary ileostomy for several weeks to divert stool from the area while it heals. Marcie can't stop crying.

GEORGE, a young race-car driver. His colostomy is temporary, to give his large intestine a chance to heal after crash injuries, but that doesn't cheer him much. "How come I get such an oddball thing?" he snarls at the doctor, the nurse, and the hospital ceiling. "Bet I'm the only one...."

The more common ostomies—colostomies and ileostomies—involve the digestive tract and depend for their success on its amazing ability to adapt to change.

Everything we eat, from apple pie to zucchini, must be broken down into tiny particles and changed to simpler chemical substances which can be absorbed into the blood stream. The resulting nutrients make their way to cells throughout the body, thus providing constant fuel and materials for energy, growth, and rebuilding. This complex process of digestion takes place in the long (about 26 feet or 8 meters in an adult) twisting internal canal known as the *intestinal* or *digestive tract*, alimentary canal, or gut.

Digestion starts in the mouth, where food is chewed and enzymes in the saliva begin the process. From there, food goes via the esophagus to the stomach where churning action, different enzymes, and weak acid continue mechanical and chemical changes.

Becoming more liquid at each stage, the food proceeds into the small intestine, where substances from the liver, gall bladder and pancreas further the process, breaking down even the most exotic foods into simple sugars, amino acids, and fatty acids. To be used by the body, the digested food must pass through the walls of the small

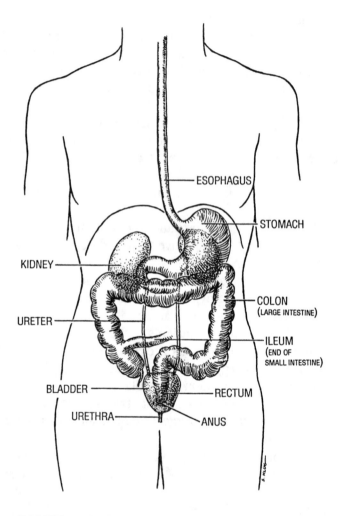

ESOPHAGUS

STOMACH

KIDNEY

COLON
(LARGE INTESTINE)

URETER

ILEUM
(END OF
SMALL INTESTINE)

BLADDER

RECTUM

URETHRA

ANUS

DIGESTIVE AND URINARY TRACTS. To make the relationships clearer, the artist has left out most of the small intestine, which twists and winds for about 20 feet (6 meters) around the abdomen of an adult, from the end of the stomach until the ileum, the last section of the small intestine, joins the large intestine (colon). The parts of the urinary tract are labeled at the left of the picture; those of the digestive tract are at the right.

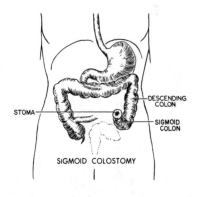

DESCENDING COLON

STOMA

SIGMOID COLON

SIGMOID COLOSTOMY

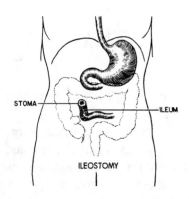

STOMA

ILEUM

ILEOSTOMY

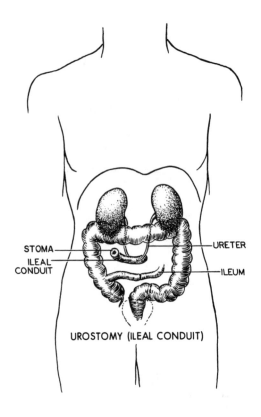

STOMA

ILEAL CONDUIT

URETER

ILEUM

UROSTOMY (ILEAL CONDUIT)

intestine by way of countless tiny fingerlike projections which line the small intestine.

By the time food reaches the colon (large intestine or large bowel), most of the nourishment and water have been absorbed. Here the major tasks are absorbing more water and some mineral salts, and transporting and storing the indigestible remains of the food in the lower part of the colon and the rectum. At the far end of the versatile winding digestive tract, the anus contains the ring-like *sphincter* muscles which open to release feces.

The digestive tract is surrounded by smooth muscles which contract and expand, mixing food with digestive juices and then propelling it from one end of the tract to the other by the rhythmic waves known as *peristalsis*. These waves are almost constant; there are also longer, slower contractions, known as mass movements, which push bowel contents into the rectum and produce the urge to move the bowels.

Usually, the whole process of digestion is so automatic and so efficient that we forget its marvelous complexity (the liver alone has over 300 functions). Once we swallow food, we don't need to think about it—unless there is a problem.

Occasionally, there is a massive breakdown in the system. The intestine may be blocked, completely or partially, by cancer, injury, or birth defect. Or food may rush through the digestive tract so quickly that there is little chance for nutrients to be absorbed; in severe inflammatory bowel disease, the person may be starving. In all these cases, an ostomy may become necessary.

The body adjusts quite nicely to a shortened digestive tract. If the ostomy occurs near the end of the digestive tract, as in a permanent colostomy, the person has lost only a storage area, and sphincters to release feces. If the ostomy is farther up in the digestive tract, as it is in some temporary colostomies and in ileostomies, the person has also lost part of the ability to absorb water, bile salts and minerals; the discharge tends to be less formed. But the remaining intestine eventually takes over some of this water-absorbing function, and the kidneys, the major regulators of water and minerals for all people, with or without ostomies, handle the rest of the adjustment.

Colostomies account for 75% of all abdominal outlet ostomies. Since colorectal cancer, the most common cause for a permanent colostomy, usually occurs in people over 50, and since it causes little or no distress in its early stages, most people who undergo colostomy surgery are over 50, and are surprised and shocked by what's being done.

There's been no warning, or only such subtle hints as a change in bowel pattern, excessive gas, or a trace of blood in the stool.

In contrast, people who have ileostomies (which account for perhaps 10 to 15% of all ostomies) tend to be teenagers or young adults, and they've often had plenty of warning. Most have had a long or unusually severe bout with a fiery dragon of a bowel. Inflammatory bowel disease has laid them low with severe diarrhea (often bloody), cramps, and weight loss. In many of these cases, an ileostomy represents an instant cure. The colon has been a battlefield; without it, peace is probable.

The final 10% of ostomies are urostomies, also called urinary diversions, since they divert, or reroute, the urine from its ordinary path. (While all urostomies are urinary diversions, there are some kinds of urinary diversions which don't result in stomas.) After the kidneys have filtered wastes out of the blood, they flush excess fluid and wastes as urine through two narrow tubes (ureters) to an expandable storage area (the bladder) and then out of the body through the urethra. At least some kidney function is essential for life, but any other part of the urinary tract can be removed or bypassed. Because reasons for urostomies vary from birth defects to cancer of the bladder, the age range here is wide, and many different surgical techniques are used.

In any abdominal outlet ostomy, the damaged, diseased, or non-working section of intestine or urinary tract is removed (or no longer used). To provide for the essential elimination of feces or urine, a new exit must be made.

For a permanent colostomy or a standard ileostomy, the surgeon tunnels the end of the remaining intestine through the muscle, fat, and skin of the abdominal wall, rolls the end over on itself like the neck of a turtleneck sweater, and stitches this in place.

The commonest permanent urostomy is called an *ileal*

conduit, not to be confused with an ilesotomy, which is for feces. To make an ileal conduit, the surgeon cuts a short section of the ileum (still attached to its blood and nerve supply) away from the rest of the small intestine, closes it at one end, and brings the open end through the abdominal wall as a stoma. The narrow tubes leading from the kidneys are connected to the section of the ileum, so that urine has a conduit, or passageway, out of the body. Finally, the remaining ends of the intestine are reconnected and resume their function of moving feces out of the body. A similar surgery which uses a section of the colon rather than the ileum is called a *colonic conduit.*

The stoma which results from any of these ostomies could be described as a soft valve. It stretches to permit waste to be expelled. During inactive periods, the tissue pulls together, rather like puckered lips (stoma, in fact, means "mouth"). Although it expands and contracts, the stoma does not have the firm muscle control of the anal or urinary sphincter; voluntary control of bowel movements or urination must be replaced by something else.

For many people with ostomies, a pouch (also called an appliance or a bag) is that "something else." This is a commercially-made pouch, usually of thin flexible plastic, which is placed over the stoma and adhered to the skin to hold feces or urine until a convenient time for disposal. An alternative chosen by many people with colostomies is *irrigation*, a kind of enema through the stoma, which permits them to empty the bowel at their convenience. They wear only a soft pad or a very small appliance over the stoma.

One variation on either the ileostomy or the ileal conduit is the *continent ostomy*, in which part of the intestine is fashioned into a reservoir inside the abdomen. This internal pouch connects to the skin via a narrow tube made of small intestine; the stoma which results is tiny, and level with the skin. The ostomy is "continent," which means that the feces or urine stays inside where it belongs, because of a valve the surgeon constructs at the outlet of the reservoir.

To manage a continent ostomy, the person inserts a plastic or rubber tube into the reservoir a few times a day to drain the feces or urine.

*****

Even though the view through a post-operative pouch may be a bit foggy, that first look at a new stoma in full, living color can be a real shocker.

In a note from Phoenix, Hazel Weathers wrote: "I wish someone had told me the stoma would be red. Red is the color usually associated with a sore or something un-healed. Although I did not have a great deal of trauma about the colostomy (I know you can't compromise with cancer), the first time I saw this stoma, I thought, 'My God, what did they do to me?' But it is now as much a part of me as my nose, ears or right hand."

Although the stoma usually shrinks somewhat in diameter as post-operative swelling goes away and normal diet and exercise resume, it remains red and moist. This is logical, since this new exit is still a part of the intestine, lined with essentially the same kind of soft velvety mucous membrane as the mouth. In fact, if the stoma changes color, and becomes blue, gray, or anything but red or deep pink, it's not getting the blood supply it needs. This happens sometimes during the first few days after surgery and requires immediate medical attention.

Unlike an incision, a stoma requires little healing. The stitches used are often the kind that don't need to be removed. A urostomy stoma starts to expel urine imme-diately, even before the patient has left the operating room; the other types of stomas start discharging feces in a few days.

CONSTRUCTING A STOMA. The cut end of the intestine is brought through the abdomen, turned back on itself and stitched to the skin.

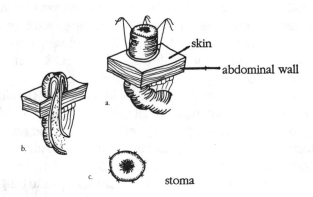

skin

abdominal wall

a.

b.

c.

stoma

Stomas come in many shapes and sizes, depending on the kind of ostomy—and the person who owns it. The stoma for an ileostomy, since it's made from the small intestine, is ordinarily smaller in diameter than a colostomy stoma, constructed from the large intestine. Some stomas are smaller than a dime in diameter; others, usually with temporary ostomies, may be much larger across.

Shape varies as much as size. Some are round, some oval, and others are irregular in shape. Most stomas protrude slightly above the abdominal wall, perhaps 1/4 to 1/2 an inch (6–13 mm). Where drainage is more constant, as is the case with urostomies and ileostomies, the stoma is usually longer. From 3/4 to one inch (about 2 cm) is said to be the ideal length. This length helps the stoma discharge waste directly into a pouch, instead of letting it pool on the skin.

At first, it's a temptation to feel over-protective about

one's stoma, feeling it's so fragile it might be damaged by a breeze in the shower. While reasonable protection is essential, the stoma is surprisingly tough. It's not harmed by water, during sexual contact, or even by gentle bumps against furniture. It doesn't have sensory nerves so is insensitive to pain. It does bleed easily, however, even from as little cause as an overzealous swipe with a wash cloth, because many tiny blood vessels are very close to its surface. A pouch or a soft pad will protect it from the friction of clothes.

Some stomas are constructed in the best possible location; others are not. Ideally, the ET nurse or the surgeon (singly or together) spends time with the patient before surgery, watching how the shape of the abdomen changes when the person is sitting, standing, bending, or walking—where the waistline is, where valleys and bulges occur. Then the probable site is marked.

If possible, the stoma is centered on a smooth and relatively flat plane, away from old scars or bones that protrude. Not all abdomens are ideal, however. Sometimes, because of fat or scars, there isn't any really good location for the stoma. And even with advance planning, the surgeon may change the site because of conditions discovered during the operation.

Within a few months after surgery, the stoma should settle down to a fairly consistent size, shape, and color. The shape may vary a little with change of position or activity, even coughing. Weight loss or gain (pregnancy, for example) may alter the contour of the stoma. But, different as stomas are from person to person, an individual stoma should look about the same from day to day, year to year. If the color changes much after the first few weeks, the stoma is probably being pinched by a too-small pouch opening; any color change that doesn't get back to normal quickly when the pouch is removed needs to be seen promptly by the doctor.

All intestinal stomas secrete some mucus, a thick liquid which helps lubricate and protect the intestine. As surplus mucus is discharged, it serves as a natural cleaning agent for the stoma. In addition, both stoma and the skin around it thrive on showers and baths, free of a pouch. (Water doesn't get into the stoma.) The stoma should not be scrubbed, however.

People vary in their wish or need to nickname the new exit. In some families, the doings of Charlie, Rosebud, or Oscar are a shared joke. Margot Julian, RN, ET, has some questions about the practice. She feels nicknames depersonalize the fact and may interfere with accepting the change. "Does one name one's foot?" she asks.

On the other hand, few feet develop such distinct personalities as stomas do. In addition to their regular functions, they sometimes whimper softly, or sigh with unexplained contentment.

Especially at first, stomas may star in dreams or fantasies. This too, is "normal." It may help one work out feelings that cannot always be shared.

This takes a while. Margot continues: "It seems like something that's been stuck on you, but it's been a part of you all your life. This is just the first time you've ever been able to see it. Sometimes it takes a while to think of it as part of yourself."

In the 18th and the 19th centuries, ostomies carried very high risks. With no anesthetics or antibiotics, patients clenched their fists and recited the 23rd Psalm. Mortality was high. With newer techniques, surgical and post-operative risks are greatly reduced, especially when surgery is done promptly.

Although grouped under common headings, no two ostomies are exactly alike—each is a very personal thing. There are some new habits to learn but that's a small enough price to pay for an improved or extended life.

CHAPTER 3 ✻ *It's Your Body*

*Sometimes good things happen in odd
ways. About 6:30 that second morning in
the hospital, I got mad—angry enough to
weep and holler and, somewhat erroneously,
call the surgeon a male chauvinist pig.*

The trouble started because I didn't feel I'd been
accurately informed about a certain diagnostic procedure.
Although I wasn't exactly proud of weeping like a
frustrated four-year-old, that early morning storm served
a purpose. After it, my surgeon and his colleagues took
greater care explaining just what was happening, and why.
Bit by bit, I became a functioning member of my treatment
team.

Despite an early tonsillectomy and having a baby, my
knowledge of hospital procedures was sketchy. However,
I knew I had some responsibility for my own body.
Yet—unless I knew what was going on—how could I
accept any part of that responsibility? What were they
doing, and why? What would the results be? What were
the risks? The discomforts? Did I have any choices?

Fortunately, my sense of personal responsibility
coincided with great changes sweeping the health care
fields. For many reasons, old ideas about physicians and

surgeons as remote and omnipotent beings whose slightest word is Holy Writ, and compliant, quavering patients with a vocabulary limited to "Yes, doctor" are being replaced by something much more like a partnership—to everyone's benefit.

Doctors, nurses, and patients are becoming more aware of patients' rights *and* responsibilities, and of the very real contribution we patients can make to our own healing. In part, this change results from a better-informed lay public and greater emphasis on patient education, in part from the impetus of the holistic health movement, and in part from the medical profession's growing awareness of malpractice hazards. These forces, along with some intangibles, have resulted in the age of informed consent.

For a long time we've known that patient attitudes may have a crucial effect on the healing process. That brave young fellow in room 517 on Ward E who makes it despite the odds is almost a cliche of novels and TV dramas; actually, such stories have a firm basis in fact and appear more and more often in the medical literature. Not all cures can be traced to Wonder Drug X. The individual who wants to live has the best chance of doing just that and, even with the best medical care, the patient's contribution—positive or negative—can make a difference.

Flora, one of our friends, happens to have two ostomies, a urostomy and a colostomy, plus other health problems. She's an active and glowing woman; she is also a trained UOA visitor, a volunteer with an ostomy who visits people shortly before or after their ostomy surgery, passing along the news that a good life is possible after an ostomy. A few months ago, she was called to visit a woman scheduled to have ostomy surgery the following week. Unfortunately, despite Flora's obvious well-being and happiness, the patient muttered, "I'd rather die than have that happen to me." She got her wish: She died on the operating table.

While there may have been other factors involved, we believe that her unwillingness to take a chance on the proposed change, her reluctance even to try life with an ostomy, may have had quite a bit to do with her premature death.

Major surgery is scarcely a do-it-yourself project, and ostomies are major surgery. I didn't have the knowledge to order the necessary tests, nor the expertise to interpret them, but I could listen. I couldn't scrub for surgery or do a physical examination, but I could say "yes," "no," "maybe," "why is this test necessary?"—or even "I'd like a second opinion."

The patient's rights to information and a certain level of care have been spelled out in a *Patient's Bill of Rights,* presented by the American Hospital Association and reprinted after this chapter.

The brave words in the Patient's Bill of Rights form a good working beginning for a team approach. They are honored more by some hospitals and physicians than by others. Some still prefer the old way and far too many patients throw away their right to know what's happening, letting the medical profession carry all the responsibility. Sometimes, though, they mutter to themselves, a roommate, a visiting spouse or friend, "I don't know what's going on. No one tells me anything." But they don't ask—and that's plum crazy.

Along with the right to ask questions goes the right to receive clear answers in words the patient knows and understands. From asking what's happening and what it means, or listening when an explanation is offered, it's not such a long step to asking sometimes, "What can I do to help?" or even, "I wonder if we could try. . . ." Participating doesn't mean constant demanding or gluing one's finger to the call bell, but it does mean awareness and some positive effort.

For the person awaiting ostomy surgery, the treatment

team seems almost as big as the production crew for a movie. (How, I wondered, could all these strangers know so much—and seem to care so much—about *my* gut?)

The team includes not only the patient (hopefully), but also the surgeon, assistants and other physicians (in a teaching hospital, where doctors spend one or more years after medical school learning under the supervision of more experienced doctors, this can mean quite a number of people). It also includes nurses. Around the clock, they're still the bulwark of treatment, including specialists who limit their services to the operating room or recovery room, as well as timid student nurses, as excited and apprehensive as you are about seeing their first ostomy.

There are also respiratory therapists, x-ray and lab technicians, dietitians, social workers, physical therapists, ward clerks, maintenance people and volunteers. Of great importance to many patients are the hospital chaplains.

Family and friends are unofficial members of the treatment team; they can help or hinder—depending in part on their level of information, in part on your rapport. However well you know each other, people are full of surprises in unexpected situations. Sometimes friends or family have unpredictable reactions, or repeat old wives' tales best forgotten. But, along with fruit, a paperback mystery and a bunch of daisies, they also bring hope.

Other patients (and their visitors) are often helpful, counteracting your anxieties with a rousing tale of what a great life their Aunt Alice has had since she had her ostomy, fifteen years ago! While hospital friendships are sometimes as brief as shipboard romances, the support and companionship of others who are not strangers to early morning temperatures and bedpans can be very heartening.

And high on the list of team members are trained visitors from the United Ostomy Association. It really helps to talk to a man, woman or child who has an ostomy—and who enjoys living.

Important, too, are both the moral support and technical know-how of an enterostomal therapy nurse (ET nurse), a specialist in how to deal with this slight change in one's plumbing. Of both UOA visitors and ET nurses, we'll have much to say later.

For any ostomy, the forecast varies—from excellent to poor (or, as they say, 'guarded'). Not all of the results are controllable. If, for instance, colorectal cancer has been discovered too late, surgery will probably result in increased comfort but not necessarily in longevity. As taboos fade, and early diagnosis becomes more the rule, earlier surgery will bring with it a brighter picture.

In any case, no matter how many big-name specialists join your treatment team, without you they're not going to make medical history. With you on the team, who knows?

PATIENT'S BILL OF RIGHTS

1. The patient has the right to considerate and respectful care.

2. *The patient has the right to obtain from his physician complete current information concerning his diagnosis, treatment and prognosis in terms the patient can be reasonably expected to understand.* When it is not medically advisable to give such information to the patient the information should be made known to an appropriate person in his behalf. He has a right to know by name the physician responsible for his care. (our emphasis)

3. The patient has the right to receive from his physician information necessary to give informed consent prior to the start of any procedure and/or treatment. Except in emergencies, such information for informed consent

should include but not necessarily be limited to the specific procedure or treatment, the medically significant risks involved and the probable duration of incapacitation. When medically significant alternatives for care or treatment exist, or when the patient requests information concerning medical alternatives, the patient has the right to such information. The patient also has the right to know the name of the person responsible for the procedures and/or treatment.

4. The patient has the right to refuse treatment to the extent permitted by law, and to be informed of the medical consequences of his action.

5. The patient has the right to every consideration of his privacy concerning his own medical care program. Case discussion, consultation, examination and treatment are confidential and should be conducted discreetly. Those not directly involved in his care must have the permission of the patient to be present.

6. The patient has the right to expect that all communications and records pertaining to his care should be treated as confidential.

7. The patient has the right to expect that within its capacity a hospital must make reasonable response to the request of a patient for services. The hospital must provide evaluation, service, and/or referral as indicated by the urgency of the case. When medically permissible a patient may be transferred to another facility only after he has received complete information and explanation concerning the needs for and alternatives to such a transfer. The institution to which the patient is to be transferred must first have accepted the patient for transfer.

8. The patient has the right to obtain information as to any relationship of his hospital to other health care and educational institutions insofar as his care is concerned. The patient has the right to obtain information as to the existence of any professional relationship between individuals, by name, who are treating him.

9. The patient has the right to be advised if the hospital proposes to engage in or perform human experimentation affecting his care and treatment. The patient has the right to refuse to participate in such research projects.

10. The patient has the right to expect reasonable continuity of care. He has the right to know in advance what appointment times and physicians are available and where. The patient has the right to expect that the hospital will provide a mechanism whereby he is informed by his physician or a delegate of the physician of the patient's continuing health care requirements following discharge.

11. The patient has the right to examine and receive an explanation of his bill, regardless of source of payment.

12. The patient has the right to know what hospital rules and regulations apply to his conduct as a patient.

No catalog of rights can guarantee for the patient the kind of treatment he has a right to expect. A hospital has many functions to perform, including the prevention and treatment of disease, the education of both health professionals and patients, and the conduct of clinical research. All these activities must be conducted with an overriding concern for the patient, and, above all, the recognition of his dignity as a human being. Success in achieving this recognition assures success in the defense of the rights of the patient.

CHAPTER 4 ✤ *Before Surgery*

> *It's good to hope. It's the waiting that spoils it.*
> Yiddish proverb

There's no such thing as a typical waiting period before ostomy surgery. Sometimes, there's no wait at all. The victim of an auto accident may end up with a temporary colostomy even before news of the crash is reported on the radio. In life-threatening situations—a woman with her bladder mangled in a car crash, or a young man with a ruptured intestine—full explanations must come after surgery. Although there's no time to explain, the news is good: The car crash victim and the young man are alive, not dead.

For others, waiting seems endless. A person who has ulcerative colitis may have had miserable months or years to get ready, while one drug after another and one treatment after another were tried. By the time surgery is finally scheduled, such patients are often eager for the freedom it promises.

I had nine days—a weekend at home and a week in the hospital—to get used to the idea of a colostomy. It was a double adjustment: both to the coming surgery and to the unexpected cancer that made it necessary.

If I'd lived closer to the hospital, many of the tests and some of the other preparation might have been done before I was admitted, since I was basically healthy and didn't need the kind of building up which some people need after a siege of severe bowel disease. (Now, almost everyone is admitted to the hospital either the day before or the morning of surgery, with much of the testing and other preparation already behind them.)

That weekend was dizzy and out of focus. Besides packing things I didn't need, and watering water-logged plants while neglecting bone-dry ones, I phoned people, saw them, went out to dinner, wrote maudlin heart-in-the mouth letters (and a last will and testament), explaining what little I knew. Although I rattled off the words like a parrot, I still didn't believe them. Then, and for the week that followed, I was cushioned by a strange sense of unreality. Surely I was only a stand-in; all the things they were talking about were really going to happen to someone else.

Driving back home with friends Sunday afternoon, I fought the odd sensation that one tire was probably going to come off the car. When we got to the city, we discovered that one tire had been slashed almost all the way through and was seriously out of alignment! They had it fixed before they returned. I felt a little less crazy.

"Come to the hospital Monday morning by eight," Dr. Wise had invited. "Without breakfast, and without coffee."

It was an omen, and a preview. All that first week in the hospital, meals would appear on time for a day or so; then I wouldn't get a tray at mealtime.

"My food didn't come."

"Sorry, doctor's orders—there's that test."

Out in the big world, great things were happening. Athletes were arriving in Montreal for the start of the Olympics on July 17. I turned my back on the pageantry on my neighbor's TV and wondered how soon I would be able to eat after surgery. That week, my horizons were on the narrow side.

What Dr. Wise had said when he set up this elaborate charade was, "We'd like to do a few more tests." That seemed the understatement of the year. Twice daily, the doctors made their rounds. Usually, their first visit was almost before the cock crowed in the morning, and then they'd pop in again, late in the afternoon. Dr. Reinker, my surgeon, was usually accompanied by the resident working with him, Dr. Banks, and by an intern barely two weeks out of medical school, who clasped his hands behind his back and looked as solemn as he could. Sometimes other doctors came along.

After each visit, they must have sprinted back to the doctors' small cubbyhole next to the nursing station to write up another three dozen orders for tests, familiar and unfamiliar, plus all the usual routine things—blood pressure, pulse, and temperature. Amazing that they could fit them all in.

The week before, the diagnosis had been made with the help of a *sigmoidoscope*. This is a tube which, inserted into the large intestine via the anus, lets the doctor see (or "scope") the last 12 inches (30 cm) or so of the intestinal tract, which is where most colorectal cancers appear. Back then, all sigmoidoscopes were rather rigid tubes; now, the doctor may use a flexible sigmoidoscope, which curves around the bends of the digestive tract more easily.

Now the doctors wanted to look at the large intestine beyond the rectum and the sigmoid colon, and that meant examination with a *colonoscope*. This flexible instrument provides a view of the entire colon, so well lighted that slides or movies can be taken if needed. Doctors can also use a colonoscope for minor colon surgery, perhaps removing a polyp or snipping a piece of tissue for a biopsy.

With either the sigmoidoscope or the colonoscope, the doctor wants to be able to see the lining of the bowel plainly, without any stool in the way. Thus, the unbeloved but necessary bowel "prep": a day or two of dwindling diet along with laxatives and/or enemas.

That was Tuesday. On Thursday, after a brief starvation diet and more laxatives and enemas than I cared for, I was introduced to the *barium enema* and the *intravenous pyelogram*. The barium enema, which seemed to involve quarts of pale, pink, liquid plaster inserted through the anus, fills the colon and makes a shadow picture of its twists and turns, together with any irregularities. X-rays are taken at various points in the barium's journey.

If the barium is swallowed rather than inserted through the anus, the films will show the outline of the gastrointestinal (GI) tract from the esophagus through the small intestine. These x-rays are called an *upper GI series* with small bowel follow-through and can provide essential information when the diagnosis is inflammatory bowel disease. (After any barium x-rays, doctors may order a laxative and/or enema to get rid of the barium before it can solidify in the intestine: It not only looks like plaster, but hardens like it.)

To complete the map of my interior, I underwent an *intravenous pyelogram* (IVP or *excretory urography*), involving a "contrast" liquid injected into an arm vein. The liquid travels through the kidneys and the rest of the urinary tract, and makes the whole tract show up clearly on x-rays, highlighting any malfunction and showing where kidneys and bladder are in relation to the colon and other landmarks. This test is relatively painless except for a brief but fiery heat flash following the injection. For those few people who are allergic to the injected substance, other tests can be used to provide the necessary information about the urinary tract.

Before urinary diversion surgery, there is *cystoscopy*, another scope, this one a tube inserted through the urethra into the bladder. Through the cystoscope, the doctor can take a careful look at the lining of the bladder and can remove a piece of tissue for a biopsy.

Besides these old standby tests, there are newer procedures like *CT (computed tomography)* and *MRI (magnetic resonance imaging)*, which give clear cross-sectional images of body parts that can't be seen well with standard x-rays. These tests involve lying still for an hour or so, sometimes after drinking or having a vein injection of a contrast material.

The CT scanner rotates around the patient, taking images from different angles, which a computer then assembles into pictures. For the MRI, the patient is wheeled headfirst into a long tube; the patient hears loud clicking noises as the computer collects data.

CT and MRI are often used to "see" the urinary tract. They don't picture the intestines well (the constantly-moving intestinal tract won't stay still for the test), but can show the quieter organs near the bowel.

With any gaps in time filled with an electrocardiogram (EKG or ECG) to check heart function, and with more blood and urine tests to show how well my liver, kidneys, and lungs were functioning, the tests were coming to an end. From them, the doctors had a fair idea of how well my body would withstand the inevitable shock of surgery.

Mechanical and lab tests were only part of the endless information-gathering process. Although I'd just had a complete physical in the weeks before the malignancy was discovered, this was a teaching hospital, so I gave my history to a seemingly endless stream of eager listeners. I told about my illnesses, allergies and lifestyle. Since all the doctors and nurses who questioned me had slightly different points of view and asked different questions, it was not pure repetition, although some days it seemed like overkill, as doctors poked and palpated, listened with a stethoscope, tested reflexes. . . .

There were some visitors, many cards, letters, and calls. Since my friend Irv had come to visit me the night I arrived, and told me the important thing about his colostomy just by being there, alive and healthy, I didn't think of requesting a UOA visitor before surgery, though I might have welcomed one. Many patients, not knowing an Irv, are dubious about seeing anyone with an ostomy before surgery, although it can be very reassuring. Judy Greaves of Coos Bay, Oregon, suggests: "The pre-op patient, waiting for this unknown, mysterious thing to happen to him, is too blamed scared to consent to anything. . . .[But] the result will be less fear of the unknown, because the patient has seen an apparently 'normal' person doing things he has always done and looking like everyone else. A short, pleasant visit by this stranger he thought of as 'mutilated' can do wonders for his morale. . . ." It could have helped.

From Monday afternoon, when the doctors came in and saw me enjoying a cigarette, there was heavy pressure to cut out cigarettes, at least for the present. As they explained it, if I stopped smoking, even for a few days, the irritation and mucus production in my lungs would decrease, and I would have a better chance of sailing through surgery and the days after without lung problems.

Their arguments moved me, and I did cut down drastically—from two packs a day to two or three cigarettes a day! (Now most hospitals are smoke-free; the smoker has to go to a special smoking area for a cigarette.)

I was helped in cutting down by the respiratory therapist who talked more about the heavy load surgery puts on the lungs and the blood stream. She brought me an engaging toy with a serious purpose, an incentive spirometer. When I put the tube in my mouth and took a really deep breath, three bright cheerful blue balls would rise to the top of their respective plastic columns. The deeper and steadier the breath, the longer they would stay at the top. Do it every hour, she suggested, but I was fascinated by this simple proof of progress in breathing, and sometimes tucked in an extra session.

I think my three roommates, a fascinating and ever-changing group (since most of them were in for minor surgery), envied me my breathing toy. I was frankly jealous of their meals, as mine petered out to nothing. There was a last bland meal on Friday night—chicken broth, baked halibut, asparagus cuts, and orange cake with frosting—and thereafter only clear liquids.

On Saturday, when I began a clear liquid diet, it seemed as if they gave me a laxative every two hours. It wasn't really that often, but I'd definitely begun the period of bowel "prep" which precedes surgery of the bowel, as well as urinary diversion surgeries which use a piece of intestine. (This prep is like that administered before a colonoscopy, but sometimes even more thorough.)

To prevent post-operative infections, and to have a clear field for surgery, surgeons, nurses, and dietitians work together to clean out the bowel; their purpose is to have the entire colon as clean as if they'd turned the hose on it. Not only any remnants of feces, but also as many as possible of the bacteria (friendly and unfriendly) which usually live in the colon, must be removed. The measures employed seem somewhat drastic to the patient.

During the "prep" there is a progression from a low-fiber diet to clear liquid, and there's an increasing concentration on laxatives and then enemas. The specifics vary from doctor to doctor, from hospital to hospital, and even from time to time. When I was getting ready for the barium enema, I'd had the dubious treat of bubble-gum flavored castor oil; a couple of months later, when I had another barium enema as a post-operative check, it had been replaced by something slightly less revolting.

These days, often the bowel prep simply involves drinking a large jug of a special solution, one cup every ten minutes, which makes a clean sweep of the intestines and usually eliminates the need for enemas. Hard as it is to drink so much so quickly, it is essential: It is the presence of such a large amount of solution in the digestive tract at one time that makes this prep work so well.

Since this kind of bowel prep wasn't available then, I had (according to a brief note I made) a laxative, five enemas and three showers on the day before surgery! These were not the relatively simple do-it-yourself Fleets prepackaged enemas, but the old-fashioned kind, administered by a determined nurse. In addition, just in case any bacteria escaped this all-out onslaught, there were several doses of antibiotic pills.

The Saturday and Sunday before surgery were marked by other highlights. People kept coming in and introducing themselves. "Hi, I'm one of the recovery-room nurses, so you'll recognize a familiar face when you wake up in the recovery room." "Hello, I'll be giving your anesthesia, and I wonder if you have any questions."

The day before surgery, Dr. Reinker took me into his office, explained just what they would be doing and, after considering my body sitting, standing, bending and lying, marked the probable site of the stoma with a brown felt-tip pen. In some hospitals, an ET nurse would have done this, or at least participated. (I didn't know it then, and he probably didn't either, but he had made a fine beginning on the *Ostomate Bill of Rights,* reprinted at the end of this chapter.)

I was overcome by strange longings, almost like those of pregnancy. In the middle of that endless day, with nothing but clear liquids sloshing around in me, I spotted Dr. Banks and made a solemn request. If my daughter would just bring me some salted soda crackers, could I lick the salt off them? We had an earnest discussion of this important though silly question. Finally, he decided he could trust me not to swallow a crumb and agreed, giving me a hug as he did so.

Though there was no time wasted on meals that last day, it was busy, between all the enemas and the three showers. I've never quite understood the rationale for those!

There'd been unmentioned highlights all week long, together with my complaining. My daughter Kerry and my son-in-law Art came in often, though I couldn't have chosen a worse week for them, given their hectic schedules. Michael Wise, the doctor who'd found the cancer, slipped in frequently, just to talk a little.

I'd brought *Walden* along, thinking I might share some beautiful thoughts with Henry David Thoreau that week, but usually I was mired thigh-deep in trivia. Still, it was a comfort to know I had a good book with me, should I need it.

And if I'd opened it, I might have chuckled at passages like this, curiously appropriate to the last day before surgery: "Simplify, simplify. Instead of three meals a day, if it be necessary eat but one; instead of a hundred dishes, five; and reduce other things in proportion."

That might have been a good thought while drifting off to sleep, following the fairly-heavy sedative Sunday night. That or: ". . . what danger is there if you don't think of any?"

OSTOMATE BILL OF RIGHTS

The Ostomate shall:

1. be given pre-op counseling.
2. have an appropriately positioned stoma site.
3. have a well constructed stoma.
4. have skilled post-operative nursing care.
5. have emotional support.
6. have individual instruction.
7. be informed on the availability of supplies.
8. be provided with information on community resources.
9. have post-hospital follow-up.
10. benefit from team efforts of health care professionals.
11. be provided with information and counsel from the ostomy association and its members.

CHAPTER 5 ❖ *Surgery, and*
                    Just After

Recovery room nurses are used to receiving a lot
of flak from woozy patients—and abject
apologies a week or two later.

Some people who undergo ostomy surgery are old pros at after-surgery rituals. I was a novice, a reluctant and even faintly belligerent newcomer to the aftermath of abdominal surgery. In theory, I might still be a member of my treatment team; in practice, I was on the bench for a time.

The last thing I remember, after the pre-op shots and the journey to the operating room on a rolling stretcher, was lecturing a masked figure in green who was shaving my lower abdomen in some surgical anteroom.

"Why did you wait till the last minute?" I asked, a little fuzzily. "When I had toe surgery [twenty-five years before], they shaved my leg the night before—all the way to the hip, painted it with Merthiolate, and then wrapped it in a pillowcase so it wouldn't get dirty."

"We do it here in the surgical area right before the operation to decrease the number of skin bacteria."

How clever, I thought, and fell asleep.

The next thing I remember was waking up in the recovery room, hours after surgery.

Now lovely chunks of sleep were interrupted by torture. Someone—a nurse I supposed—kept waking me up.

"Take a deep breath and cough."

"I can't."

"Yes, you can. Breathe deep now, and cough."

She seemed not only mean but stupid. Didn't she know that sleep is the great healer? That gentle sleep is nature's soft nurse?

If only they'd stop nagging and leave me alone! I'd nod off and then another voice would cut in, "Come on, now, you have to take a deep breath and cough."

Yet, underneath this running battle with the nurses, an odd awareness surfaced from time to time. For better or for worse, surgery was over. And I was alive. It wasn't a constant thought—but it was magic when it came.

There are, I discovered, good reasons for those painful and seemingly endless commands during the first few days after surgery—*take a deep breath and cough.* Following the advice helps prevent lung complications.

No one longs for the not-so-good old days when a bullet to bite on and a jigger of rum sustained people through surgery. General anesthesia, which makes possible deep unconsciousness during an operation, has revolutionized surgery. However, anesthetics make great demands on the body, especially the lungs. Anesthetics irritate the lining of the lungs; these, in response, produce extra mucus to soothe the irritation. The anesthetic also paralyzes the tiny hairs in the respiratory tract which normally sweep mucus out of the lungs. If the mucus isn't removed, it clogs the air sacs in the lungs so they can't inflate with air. The temporarily-collapsed air sacs become warm, moist havens for bacteria.

Energetic and frequent coughing and deep breathing

help loosen and bring up mucus so the airway remains free. Coughing is more comfortable if a patient hugs a pillow or two tightly over the abdominal incision. This splints the wound and reduces the fear that the stitches or staples will pop open. They won't, even without a pillow.

In the post-surgery recovery room, oxygen is routinely given to help the lungs after anesthesia; it also can speed wound healing. Electrodes on the chest, hooked up by wires to a heart monitor, trace the heart's activity on a screen. Again, this is usually a routine precaution, not a sign of crisis. (Some hospitals encourage people waiting for surgery to visit the recovery room before the operation so they'll know what to expect.)

The next morning, back in my own room, I watched an eager young nurse waltz in.

"How are you feeling, Mrs. Mullen?"

I didn't answer.

"It's time to walk now."

Walk! They were out of their minds. It hurt too much just to turn over in bed. But I walked, lurching and hurting.

It was a nurse, John, who taught me the secret of moving more comfortably. "OK, now, before you try to turn over, take a deep breath and let it out slowly as you turn. You can't tense your muscles while you're expelling your breath." Absurd and simple-minded though his remedy sounded, it worked, not only for turning over but for getting out of bed. And walking.

As it turns out, there are excellent reasons for walking, as for coughing. Lying in bed too long can cause problems after surgery. When people lie down, their lungs don't expand as well as they do during standing or walking. In addition, blood tends to slow down on its return to the heart, and may form small clots. To prevent these and other bad effects of prolonged bedrest, patients walk, willingly or unwillingly. If one is available, a wheelchair to push makes a dandy companion for those first strolls outside the room: a steady support when walking—and a convenient seat if needed.

All of this walking and turning and coughing becomes much easier if one takes enough pain medicine (analgesics, often narcotics) during the first few days after surgery. Many people are nervous about taking narcotics after surgery for pain relief, but this does *not* lead to drug addiction and does help patients get better sooner—becuase they *can* walk and cough and thus avoid complications. At first, pain medication is given by injection into the muscle, under the skin, or through the vein. Instead of having to wait for a nurse, many patients can push a button on their own Patient-Controlled Analgesia (PCA) pump and deliver a small, measured dose of pain medicine through the vein. Medicine can be given by mouth after the digestive tract starts working again.

I'd been so busy defending myself against all these orders that I hadn't paid much attention to my new status as a porcupine. Back in my room, I saw that there was a tube in my hand, another in my nose, and one going into the bladder. Each tube was attached to something on the outside.

I'd expected the intravenous (IV) line, for I'd had one before. This tube, inserted directly into a vein, serves as a life-line, making possible the swift administration of blood, fluids, medicines, and short-acting anesthetics. The IV tube hangs from a plastic pouch or a glass bottle, full of fluids, suspended on a portable stand. From a patient's viewpoint, the IV has great nuisance value. If I walked, it went along.

I had not expected the tube which went through my nose and down the esophagus to the stomach (irritating my throat along the way). As a rule, the intestinal tract goes into hibernation for a few days after abdominal surgery. This tube, called a nasogastric or NG tube, is connected to a suction machine to remove gas and stomach secretions. Without the help of this small tube, these can build up, cause acute discomfort and perhaps vomiting, and put strain on the fresh surgical stitches. Sometimes there's no need for an NG tube; other times an NG tube may be used for a day or even several days. (Instead of inserting a tube through the nose, some surgeons place a similar tube through a small slit in the skin into the stomach—a gastrostomy tube—or another part of the digestive tract; this, connected to suction, performs the same functions of keeping the patient comfortable and protecting the surgical site. The slit heals quickly after the tube is removed.)

Sore throat, a common complaint after any major surgery, is often caused by another tube, this one inserted through the mouth into the lungs after the person is asleep in the operating room and removed before the person wakes up. This tube delivers the long-lasting anesthetic into the lungs and makes breathing easier during the operation.

Finally, there was a catheter (tube) inserted directly into the bladder to drain urine into an external bag which hung on the side of my bed. The bladder, inevitably pushed around some during abdominal surgery, may turn sluggish for a time. The external collection bag allows staff to check the urine output. It's also convenient not to have to worry about wet beds or coping with a bedpan when sitting and moving are still such painful, risky business.

So, when I walked I had company: the IV stand, the temporarily-disconnected NG tube, and the somewhat embarrassing bag of urine. No one paid any attention.

Like many people with new ostomies, I was in no hurry to survey the alterations to my anatomy. Since the digestive system has slowed to a halt, the person with an ileostomy or a colostomy can ignore the stoma for a few days after surgery. One sneaks a look—it is there, red and foreign, inside the plastic post-op pouch, but it isn't doing much and it doesn't hurt.

The incision does hurt. There's a glimpse of that, too, when the dressing is changed. For many patients with a permanent colostomy or ileostomy, the most painful sensations come from a wound one can't see—the large opening where the rectum and anus used to be. This wound, which can make sitting uncomfortable for weeks to come, is treated in different ways by different surgeons.

The person with a new urostomy, on the other hand, cannot ignore the new stoma. With the bladder removed or disconnected, urine discharge is constant, from the minute the stoma is constructed on the operating table. On the other hand, the rectum and anus aren't removed so there is no uncomfortable rear wound.

I tried to catch up.

"Why didn't the doctor come and see me in the recovery room after surgery?" I asked my daughter.

"He did—three times. Doctor Wise came too. And so did I."

"Really? That's nice." I said it as politely as I could, knowing that she was kidding me. If they'd come, surely I would have remembered?

But maybe not. There was a big blank spot when I couldn't have remembered if a bagpipe corps had come and serenaded me (that would have been nice). The memory blank results from the aftereffects of anesthesia, fairly heavy pain and sleep medication in the first few days after surgery, and perhaps the body's intuitive need to protect itself from pain.

I think I asked the same questions dozens of times.

"How long was I in surgery?"

"About four hours."

"Did I have any transfusions?"

"Yes, four units of blood."

"The tumor—was it really malignant?"

"Yes."

"Did you get it all?"

"We hope so."

Everyone has a different experience in surgery. Too, everyone reacts differently. We differ in our tolerance for pain and/or discomfort, the speed with which we heal, the swiftness with which we wake up after surgery, and many other things. And though some patterns may seem luckier than others, no one way is right. . .

In spite of my grumbles, I was lucky. Thanks to those nagging nurses (and a basically healthy body), there were no major post-op complications. And people had come to see me, even if I didn't remember them.

For most patients, the days just after surgery tend to be foggy. One is not always rational or logical. Still, with much help from nursing staff, family and friends, most of us manage to muddle through.

The surgery had taken place Monday morning. On Thursday, the doctor was delighted when my system started a noisy rumbling. That meant my body was beginning to take over its own chores again, and so the NG tube could go. I could eat and drink, even though that first meal—apple juice, chicken broth, and lemon jello—was not much of a reward.

But I was alive. Alive and beginning to hope.

So—when I ran into the recovery-room nurse waiting for the elevator, I apologized for calling her a bitch.

CHAPTER 6 ❄ *On the Mend*

Learn the lines and get on with it.
Spencer Tracy

With the tubes out, pain medication cut down, and solid food promised (if not yet delivered), it was time to open my eyes and really look at the changes surgery had made.

It would also have been a good time to remember the Serenity Prayer, but I'm not sure that I did:

SERENITY PRAYER

God grant me the serenity
to accept the things I cannot change,
the courage to change the things I can,
and the wisdom to know the difference.

At the time, my biggest problem was that last line, "the wisdom to know the difference." One of these days, surely, everything would be put back together the way it was supposed to be?

In a more realistic mood, I realized I couldn't change the stoma, but I could get acquainted with it, perhaps teach it manners, or even show it who was boss.

I couldn't change the wound where my rectum and anus used to be; however, back now to a normal diet and a little more exercise, perhaps I could speed its healing.

As for the incision, already it was losing its angry, primitive look. It was possible, I supposed, that a normal diet and walking might help that heal too.

Everything hinged on a normal diet, but that was not quite as simple as I hoped. My mind had dreamed of real food; my body, though hungry, seemed less adventurous. It was as if my stomach had gotten so used to doing without, it had no intention of doing with.

I looked at the chicken broth and balked, feeling queasy. I looked at the lemon jello and felt small waves of nausea. How was I ever going to get strong again if even looking at food. . .? After a day or so of discomfort, I remembered an old folk remedy for nausea: ginger. Please, I asked my daughter, get me some gingersnaps.

As a matter of fact, the gingersnaps, taken in tiny bites with sips of milk, worked. Twenty-four hours later, I was ready to begin to eat. The truth is, though, that twenty-four hours later I might have been ready to begin to eat, with or without the gingersnaps. It simply takes a little time for the body, spoiled by instant if scanty nourishment via an IV tube, to start working again. And one proceeds slowly. Chicken broth, then bland, hot cereal, then—maybe—a bit of roast chicken.

In retrospect, my impatience with this minor delay in returning to normal is absurd. Many people recovering from any major surgery (including ostomy surgery) must proceed a great deal more slowly than I did. Many start with soft, bland diets, once they graduate from liquids, and inch their way slowly up the ladder again—one food at a time.

With the return of "real" food, the stoma can no longer be ignored. It begins to work, spasmodically, almost whimsically. Odd rumblings and noises. And, at irregular intervals, the discharge of feces.

Referring to my stoma, nurses would ask, "How's your rosebud?" It's a nickname, but I couldn't see the resemblance. If it looked like anything, a rolled anchovy was more like it.

In most ways, my hospital was excellent, but there was no ET nurse on the staff, nor was there a nurse with special training in the care of ostomies. What's more, it was the middle of July. This meant a crop of brand new graduate nurses who were lucky if they'd seen a ten-minute film on the care of ostomies in the course of their training.

My stoma was covered with a closed-end "colostomy" pouch, which had to be discarded whenever it filled. (As I learned later, it would have been a blessing for all of us if I'd had a drainable pouch at first, one which could have stayed in place for several days and just been emptied when it filled.)

Each nurse seemed to have a different idea about how to care for my colostomy and I, not realizing that some of them were inexperienced, tried to fit all the odd pieces together. The first nurse who changed the bag made a great thing about applying tincture of benzoin after cleaning the skin. From her enthusiasm, I gathered this would protect the skin. In fact, it irritates some people's skin. Its primary function around a stoma is to provide a tackier surface so the appliance sticks more tightly. What's more, its use has declined sharply as better adhesives have been developed.

When a different nurse came to change the pouch the next day, I wasn't exactly helping, but I was supervising. "Where's the tincture of benzoin?" I demanded. "We have to have tincture of benzoin."

"We do? Why?"

I wasn't sure, really, but after some delay, she found the tincture of benzoin. It was trial and error for both of us, with inadequate information, but at least I was beginning to participate.

Soon after the other tubes came out, and the stitches, the doctor announced on his early-bird rounds that they were going to teach me to irrigate that day. Irrigation, I knew, was a special, gentle enema through the stoma so that stool would pass once every day or two when I wanted it to, and not at other times. The idea did not excite me, and it was not a good experience. Two nurses arrived with a large, old-fashioned enema bag and a large catheter. We crowded into a cold and tiny bathroom; I didn't like any part of it.

"How did the irrigating go?" the doctor asked, expecting a joyous answer.

"Badly, thank you."

The next day, we moved to a larger and warmer bathroom, and they brought a real colostomy irrigating set with a small, smooth, cone-shaped piece of plastic to fit over the end of the irrigating tube. The experience still wasn't a happy one.

"Tell you what," said the doctor, "we'll get Jean Alvers to come over and show you how to do it. She's an ET."

Jean came that night and I was cheered by her visit. She explained some of the hows and whys of irrigating. The next morning, I told the nurses I would do it myself, and I did. It was a success, but I still didn't like the process, or want to repeat it.

Irrigation is a happy choice for thousands of people with permanent colostomies. For others, including me, it is not. A strong dislike for enemas in any form (a souvenir of my childhood) had been reinforced by the bowel prep the week before surgery, and by those frustrating first attempts.

By then, I'd had a visitor from the Golden Gate Chapter of the United Ostomy Association, and she'd left me a treasure of a booklet: *Colostomies—A Guide.* Somewhere in the middle, I found this sentence: "Some people with a descending or a sigmoid colostomy find that by eating selected foods at specific intervals, they can make the bowel move at a time convenient to them."

From that day on, whenever the doctor asked about irrigation, I shook my head and showed him the book. He was, I think, a little baffled by my stubbornness, but he did say, "It's your decision."

For a pouch, I discovered by chance a makeshift one which worked reasonably well; if it was something less than ideal, at least the management of my stoma was in my own hands.

Jean Alvers had left her phone number and had encouraged me to call if there were any problems, but I hesitated to bother her. That was a mistake. If I had called, I might have learned about other secure alternatives much sooner. Those first days are the time to learn the rudiments of control: skin care, appliance choices, emptying, changing, cleaning, and all the other rituals of this new life. Many people may need or wish to change materials and methods later. The important thing in the hospital is to begin to learn a reasonably comfortable way to deal with one's stoma. (Now patients are discharged from the hospital so soon after surgery that it's often the home care nurse who teaches basic ostomy care skills.)

The doctors continued their twice-daily rounds, admiring the stoma and checking the incision. It was a beautiful stoma, the surgeon insisted. Although beautiful was not the word I would have chosen, I later discovered that it is indeed an excellent stoma, neat and of a good size.

At first, I found the doctors' constant interest in the gaping wound between my buttocks curious and mildly embarrassing, but one adjusts. And they were paying attention where it seemed appropriate. My biggest discomfort remained that pain in my butt—the *perineal* or *posterior wound.* (It's called the "perineal" wound because the incision is along the perineum, the area from behind the genitals to where the anus used to be.) It felt bruised; it was impossible to sit squarely on it. It was less pain than acute discomfort—the kind of sore, aching numbness that sometimes happens after horseback riding, without any of the pleasure.

Many people with colostomies or ileostomies have such a wound where the rectum and anus used to be, and a most peculiar wound it is. In many operations, when surgeons remove an organ, they can count on other nearby organs to fill in the cavity. Not so when rectum and anus are removed. Because of the bony structures surrounding the area, no other organs can move into the gap.

What the body does—at varying rates of speed—is to form scar tissue to fill this hole.

Surgeons have different techniques for dealing with the empty space in the meantime. A few simply leave the wound open, packing it firmly with gauze. As the wound heals from the inside out, the space gets smaller and smaller and the amount of gauze is reduced.

Some surgeons loosely baste the skin together, inserting soft drainage tubes to remove blood and other fluid by gentle suction. This was the treatment I had; soft, thick, absorbent pads were fastened loosely over the area with paper tape (a rather casual approach, it seemed to me). Drainage, heavy at first, tapers off so that smaller pads can be used.

Other surgeons close the wound with stitches placed in the deep tissues. This way the perineal wound can heal at the same rate as the abdominal wound.

Whatever the technique, it takes time for the body to create the scar tissue to fill that empty space.

Perineal wounds are mysterious in many ways. Some heal in two months or less. Others (though drainage and discomfort have decreased) may take a year or more. Occasionally it takes more surgery to get a perineal wound to heal: opening and cleaning the area, or even a plastic surgery procedure in which muscle tissue, transplanted from elsewhere in the body, helps fill in the gap.

The day after the doctor ordered three sitz baths a day for me, I wanted to hug him. Basically, a sitz bath involves sitting for 15 or 20 minutes three times a day in about six inches (15 cm) of very warm water. The heat eases soreness and relaxes muscles. It also increases blood circulation to the area, speeding healing.

My hospital had built-in sitz baths in special small rooms. More common now is the disposable sitz bath, a plastic basin large enough to sit in, which rests on the toilet bowl and is filled with very warm water. The patient can take this home and use it, or can improvise with a large plastic tub or a generous-sized baby bath tub. A full tub bath doesn't work as well, since soaking in a full bath 20 minutes three times a day saps too much energy (and uses too much water). In the hospital or at home, a thick folded bath towel on the bottom of the sitz bath or tub makes sitting easier. A dental irrigating device may also clean the wound and help it heal faster.

In the hospital, I learned to carry a bed pillow with me, wherever I walked, just in case I decided to sit down. Even then, I sat gingerly, on one buttock or the other. A square of foam rubber, three to four inches thick, makes a good portable seat. Doughnut-shaped inflated rings should not be used, since they can encourage the wound to pull apart.

Sensations in the perineal wound or the area around it differ. Many report a continuing urge to defecate in the old way; this sensation is comparable to the "phantom limb" sensation common to amputees. Although the necessary equipment is missing, the nerves are still active. Sometimes, sitting on a toilet eases the sensation, by sending a helpful message to the brain.

There are also aching and tingling sensations; these

also decrease as healing proceeds. If the pain gets much worse, if the drainage looks like pus, or if there are other signs of infection (like a fever), it's time to check with the doctor.

For the person with a new ostomy, the days in the hospital after surgery are busy, even crowded. There is so much to learn, so many different things to try to cope with.

There are other decisions to make—or at least consider.

Not long before I went home, Dr. Reinker and I talked some about the malignancy that had brought all this about. He hoped they had gotten every last cancer cell, but there had been some spread. The cancer was in several adjoining lymph nodes so these had been removed; with luck, no stray cells would be wandering around the lymphatic system.

He recommended that I consider a course of radiation, aimed at the perineal area, as a precautionary measure. (Sometimes, now, this is given before surgery, or both before and after.) The consulting doctors agreed. However, he emphasized that this would be my decision.

Chemotherapy, then, had little to offer the person with colorectal cancer. That has changed. Now, it's saving lives or extending them for many people with either colorectal or bladder cancer. It makes sense to talk with an *oncologist* (cancer doctor) about what's new and effective.

As I remember, I was so absorbed in the day-to-day details of dealing with the stoma, comforting the perineal area with sitz baths and soft cushions, and trying to move back to reality (wherever that might be), that the word *cancer* didn't really register with me. And yet I'm sure it was there, in my unconscious. At that time, I knew two people who had undergone colostomy surgery. My friend Irv, whose ostomy was temporary, was doing fine; my friend Susan was not. She'd had surgery many weeks before I had; when I was discharged and went home,

Susan was still in the hospital, and still in bed most of the time. It was scary to wonder which path I might follow.

I was supposed to be resting, taking it easy, and yet there were all these problems to face, or postpone facing. I could echo what actress Barbara Bel Geddes said of her own mastectomy: "There's no sense in saying it's a little itty, bitty thing. It was a helluva blow."

The mail brought welcome though sometimes puzzling cards and letters from friends. Helen wrote, "If anybody was prepared for what you are going through, it is you. And I'm proud of you, gal."

Prepared? How?

Proud? Why?

Although energy was returning, it was still in short supply. Relatively minor nuisances loomed like major plagues. Like many people, I developed a bladder infection as a result of the bladder catheter; this causes a desire to urinate almost constantly and a burning sensation. Fever may also be a symptom. Antibiotics and plenty of fluids are the usual treatment.

Although I sometimes wondered at her patience with my vapors, my daughter continued to be a frequent and welcome visitor. Sometimes my son-in-law or a grandchild came along. Friends and relatives cheered me with short visits, and I enjoyed talking with my roommates as well as with doctors and nurses.

Small things delighted me. The hospital had a short supply of soft, old, much-laundered gowns, and a big supply of new and stiff ones. It was a good day when a friendly nurse slipped me a soft one.

Along with mastering the here and now, there has to be some planning for the future. Here the social worker/discharge planner becomes a resource, with information about what aid may be available. For the temporarily-sidelined worker, for instance, sick leave benefits and disability insurance (private or state) may help with living expenses.

Federal Government disability payments in the U.S. come through the Social Security Administration. To receive them, one must either be totally disabled or expect to be disabled for at least one year. Most people with ostomies simply do not qualify—they'll be up and about long before a year has passed. Emergency funds may be available through General Assistance. Social workers or hospital financial counselors can guide patients through the medical bill thicket: private health insurance, Medicare, Medicaid (Medi-Cal in California), government-mandated programs for uninsured patients, and so on.

I was ambivalent about leaving the hospital, in spite of what they'd done to me. It would be great to be home again, and yet part of me savored that sheltered existence, where other people made many of the decisions—or at least did the leg work.

And—one mystery remained.

When I'd started the physical which led to finding the cancer which led to the surgery which led to the colostomy, I'd been 100% sure that I had a stomach ulcer.

Where had it gone?

CHAPTER 7   ❧ *But How Do You Really Feel?*

In the weeks after surgery, trifles seemed to bother me most—small woes standing in for bigger ones I wasn't ready to face. When the diet kitchen didn't send my milk, I swiveled into a rage. If the vending machine in the hospital canteen grabbed my quarters, giving nothing in return, I was awash with tears. And yet, when Dr. Wise asked, "How do you really feel?" I chirped "Fine!" Sometimes I was lying.

Of course positive thinking has great value, many clouds have silver linings, and we should all look at the bright side of things.

But trying to rush the Pollyanna process seldom works. We can't even see the bright side until we've allowed ourselves to really feel our sorrow. Our sorrow. Our anger. Our sense of loss. And our fear.

However we may try to kid ourselves, for most of us there's bound to be a sense of outrage when we glimpse our changed bodies after ostomy surgery, and also a nostalgic longing for the way things used to be, before all of this happened. Though our bowels or our bladders may have caused us pain, embarrassment, trouble, and even isolation for weeks or months or years, we were used to them. They were part of us, long taken-for-granted systems which had provided us with simple but constant satisfaction for more years than we could remember. Tattered and worn though the afflicted portions of our intestines or our bladders might have been, they were ours.

And now they are gone.

As Richard J. Wells, MD, said: "People still have an inordinate emotional attachment to their own organs of elimination no matter how diseased they become. They will gladly part with a gall bladder, a stomach, 90% of their liver, or even a piece of brain, but suggest removing the bladder or the rectum and the red lights begin to blink."

Sometimes that grief is irrational—a person with ulcerative colitis doesn't lose control with surgery but regains it—yet that doesn't make the sorrow any smaller. We're not always rational people. However wise and grownup we've managed to become, there's a shadow of a hurt child underneath.

But things aren't the way they used to be, and we have stomas to prove it. And that is sorrow number two. There was a reasonably nice, reasonably slender abdomen and now there's a puffy lump with an incision, plus that *thing*, all veiled in plastic. It's true the incision is healing, the puffiness is receding, and I'm long past the age for entering the Miss America contest, but still—I had this image of myself, and now it's changed.

There is also a new vocabulary. People from many cultures have been taught to be silent, at least in polite society, about excretory functions. Thus, we may wince at this new necessity of calling a spade a spade, of using blunt words like *feces* and *rectum* and *anus* instead of "the little girl's room."

There's something else. We're different now, different from most people we know. And we don't like that. Growing up, we wanted a doll like Sarah's or a bike like Jim's, and later, a car like Peter's and a house like the Smiths'. It was safer, not being different, but now we are.

That's a lot of sorrows. If we pretend they're not there, they're apt to fester and grow. However, let out of hiding, our grief and sorrow seem to run their course and dwindle down to a manageable size, so we can begin to savor life again, including the surgery which gave us a second chance. We even begin to see the funny side—sometimes.

But just as we're not always completely rational, we're not always completely honest. And there are temptations. We want medals for bravery (since we can no longer win them for going potty) and so we lie.

"How do you feel?"

"Fine and dandy."

Only we don't. We're just putting on (or trying to put on) shining faces for staff and visitors—especially family—and for ourselves. Postponing the mourning, the good cry that's a necessary step in healing. Only after tears can the funny bone become operative again.

There's also a strange and ironic emotional peekaboo in trying too hard to be brave. Close relatives and friends were also grieving—about me and for me. Their feelings were different from mine, perhaps, but no less strong: "We were sad about the changes that had happened to you and, like you, angry at whatever fate made this surgery necessary. We wanted to reach out and let you know how much we cared. Sometimes we could. Other days, you pushed us away with your smile, your jaunty reassurance that everything was fine."

Shared laughter grows but shared grief tends to shrink, exposed to air and sun. If others are grieving with you, don't work too hard to hide your tears, or force them to postpone theirs.

It's a curious thing. We don't have to recount all these sorrows to everyone, and maybe not to anyone but ourselves. What we must do, though, is recognize them. Then, though traces of sadness may continue to surface from time to time, we don't have to cry very long. I remember with thanks a nurse who not only permitted me to cry through her lunch break but encouraged me to do so.

As Victor Alterescu, RN, ET, wrote in what is now the *Journal of ET Nursing*, "What the new ostomate must begin to do then is to let go: let go of his former body image; let go of his diseased bladder or bowel; let go of the secondary gains that often accompany illness; in short, let go of all those feelings, thoughts and memories that keep him from becoming the person he is now. . . .

"It often happens that a new ostomate cannot begin this process of letting go and freeing himself. Sometimes just thinking about all that has happened is too awful. The person appears to be in despair, and despair colors the way one looks at all of reality. It is the patient's view of reality that needs scrutiny."

Looking back, I may have tried a little too hard to sidestep this process of mourning. A more honest look at how I felt in those weeks just after surgery might have prevented some black periods later.

And yet, although this necessary process of mourning these changes cannot be evaded, neither can it be pushed and hurried. Each of us brings different weaknesses—and strengths—to this encounter with reality, and a certain innate mind-body wisdom may control the timing of the confrontation.

Gertrude Ujhely, RN, says: ". . .the danger of grief does not lie in what one feels, but rather in one's inability to tolerate one's experience. . .one's blocking or repressing one's state. . .the feelings, whether accepted or not, continue to lead their own existence—if necessary, outside one's awareness."

For all of us who have ostomies because a malignancy has been discovered, there is a double-header of shock, sorrow, and fear. Cancer is still one of the big scare words, hard to accept as having any personal meaning for us. I suspect some of us spend an inordinate amount of time fussing about our stomas so we won't have a chance to look at the other—and darker—side of the coin: "Did they get it all?" "How long do I have?" "What's the use?"

Such determined pessimism doesn't leave enough room for sensible optimism and determination. Great strides have been and continue to be made in the war against cancer. With early detection, there's a reasonable chance that they did get it all. There are also still too many unknowns about "cancer," which is not just one disease but a catch-all term for more than 100 disorders!

And—there's the mysterious factor of remission. For reasons no one understands, the six months that were all a doctor could promise have a way of stretching.

When Elsie Klein of Pennsylvania was 76, a busy widow managing her own home and large garden, she noticed a change in her bowel habits. After many tests, the doctors discovered she had well-advanced cancer of the rectum. It had spread into her reproductive organs, requiring not only a colostomy but also a hysterectomy.

Her surgery was hard and convalescence slow. The doctor did not expect her to live more than six months. An excellent seamstress, she proceeded to design and make her own "funeral dress," and made other arrangements. Once she'd done what she had to, she got busy living for the present—concentrating on her flower garden, making two huge hooked rugs, getting involved with other projects and with people.

The six months passed quickly. So did one year, two, three. Six years after her surgery, her surgeon died.

Years later, still healthy, happy and alert, Elsie Klein

gave an interview when she celebrated her 92nd birthday. The "funeral dress" was still waiting for her, 16 years after surgery. She smiled when asked about the dress: "It's probably yellowed with age."

Wynn Bullock, the famous photographer, didn't go along with the idea of cancer in his future after his colostomy. When his doctor said he had only six months to live, Bullock answered, "I have too many things to do to die that soon!" He proceeded to finish some important writing projects, take a few more photographs, star in a movie about his photography, and work his way through a huge stack of projects for the next two years!

His widow, Edna Bullock, remembers that he said, "Well, having cancer, what do I want to do? Do I want to sit around and think about it? I want to think about things I'm interested in. . . .Everything we do now is constructive, and it will continue to be."

Feelings of outrage, sorrow, fear and anger are normal and getting through them—or most of them—is a necessary chore. Many people with ostomies agree that once in a while there may be a brief tweak of old sorrow popping up, even five or 10 years later. By that time, though, so many new good things have happened that the memory is usually briefer than a quick sprinkle of rain.

Some people start to take an honest look at their feelings and then are so paralyzed they don't move on through to the other side, the good side. That's really sad—when people can't see the wide horizon beyond their ostomies.

Victor Alterescu concludes, "In the long run, the rehabilitation of the ostomy patient will not depend on whether his appliance is vinyl or rubber, belted or beltless, clear or opaque. The ostomate who accepts himself, the one who has resolved his loss successfully, will be capable of meeting his appliance needs.

"The ostomate who still feels empty, depressed, angry, and ashamed, whose energy is spent trying to contain those memories from which he cannot separate himself, may not only have appliance problems, but also other physical symptoms that result from repressing so many strong feelings of loss."

Neither ET nurses, other nurses, nor doctors have unlimited time for listening and counseling, much as they might wish for elastic days. A support group (such as UOA) can help a lot. The person who does not begin to glimpse a rainbow after a month or two might consider a brief course of professional counseling—at a mental health clinic or with a psychiatrist or other therapist who understands the many complexities and mysteries of adjusting to bodily change. After all, a second chance at life is too big a bonus to waste or fritter away with worry and gloom.

CHAPTER 8 ❁ *That Strange*
Big World Out There

*Although one me was eager to get out of the
hospital, all the other me's were terrified at the
idea, and it was the cowards who had a quorum.*

Four weeks and two days before, the hospital and all
the things they were talking about doing to me there had
seemed unreal. Now, everything was topsy-turvy. It was
the "real" world that seemed strange and unreal, and the
hospital which seemed real. Of course that feeling, like
many others that would surface in the next few months,
was transient.

When I was discharged, I camped with Kerry and Art
and their family in their home near the hospital, until they
took off on a long-planned vacation (and my check-ups
stretched out to once a week). While there I slept a lot,
worried some, and made a few timid trips to the store.
Then my cousin and his wife drove me back home to
Santa Rosa, with a thoughtful stop at the supermarket to
stock up on all the things my empty apartment wouldn't
have.

A day or two later, I wrote to a friend: "With the wound

healing, I can sit better and am having small but steady quantum leaps of energy. Yesterday, friends came over and fixed dinner, washed the dishes, vacuumed but talked too late.

"I've not yet adjusted to here—forget where things are and what kind of coffee cups I have. . . ."

If I didn't know what kind of coffee cups I had, who did? Divorced for a number of years, I was used to living alone and enjoyed many parts of such a life. The process of getting back into the world again would be much different if there were a spouse waiting—possibly better, possibly worse, but certainly different.

There were good friends close by in the apartment complex who welcomed me back, yet I felt lonely after the hospital. In part, at least, this was a communication problem. I didn't want to think about my colostomy all the time (and there were longer and longer periods when I forgot all about it), but it still had a way of creeping into my mind, wanted or not.

Sometimes, with a private chuckle, I'd hear an expression like "get your shit together" and find it all too apt (had that vulgarity been coined by someone with an ostomy?). Or I would be reminded, for instance, as I figured out that the small paper-like fragments in my stool were not parchment but potato skins! In the hospital, a roommate, a nurse or a doctor would have shared the joke. However, I doubted whether any of my neighbors would be amused by such an early-morning confidence!

In a way, the joke was on me. I'd always thought discussions about bowel habits an extra-large bore and had avoided them when I could. With so many fascinating things in the world to talk about, how could anyone want to waste time talking about the virtues of a new laxative? Or share their anxiety because they couldn't get "regular?" The worst, just a few weeks before, had been someone who'd discovered the joys of coffee enemas!

And now here I was, often finding the activities of my digestive system the most fascinating topic in the world! The United Ostomy Association came to my rescue. In answer to my call, I had not one but two visitors, pronto. Ann Kaufman and Dorothy Siercks were all the things UOA visitors should be, including lots of fun (and we've been good friends ever since). Because they shared my amusement at the strange ways of stomas (not to mention their owners), the colostomy could begin to move away from center stage.

It didn't take long to find out that Ann and Dorothy were both interested in a great many things besides ostomies. Ann and her husband Ed are excellent sailors and Ann sparkled when she told about a recent day's sailing on San Francisco Bay. Dorothy and her husband, Lloyd, are tireless weekend explorers, fishing and camping all over Northern California.

When my visitors left, they gave me a wonderful stack of back issues of *Ostomy Quarterly*, the official publication of the United Ostomy Association. Even though I was plumb in the middle of an exciting mystery novel, it got shoved aside that night. Here, perhaps, were some of the answers I'd been looking for. It was good to find such an interesting group of people, thinking about some of the same big problems that worried me, and fretting about some of the same little ones.

In addition to the boost I got from Ann's and Dorothy's visit, subsequent phone calls, and UOA meetings I began to attend, the mail brought many unexpected shots in the arm, letters from old friends and letters from strangers. That happened this way: For the past two years, I'd been writing a light-hearted column for a local weekly, the *Santa Rosa News Herald*. After my surgery, David Bolling, the editor, wrote and asked: "What's it like? Painful? Inconvenient? Frustrating? Frightening?. . .What causes rectal cancer? Please don't read that as the mercenary musings of an editor incapable of talking about real life. I'm curious, vicariously afraid. . . . What the hell? Drop me some notes."

Although I was timid about giving my neighbor, Mrs. Jones, a play-by-play account of my surgery, I decided to write a relatively light-hearted column about the adventure. The response was great: letters, phone calls, even requests for help (as if six or seven weeks of trial and error made me some kind of an expert).

An old friend, Marian, wrote, "What's the big deal? My mother has had her colostomy for 17 years now, and it's never slowed her down." Remembering Marian's mother, I knew that.

A writer I knew surprised me with this note, showing an awareness of both the downs and the ups: "I have a close awareness of a colostomy, as I nursed my mother through her post-surgery with the same procedure. She, like yourself, had tremendous spirit and determination and rose above even that. When you are sharing daily a problem such as this, you realize all the ramifications.

"Also, I have another friend who is in her forties who has had an ileostomy. She was the one who encouraged me to go to the singles dances when I was widowed. We'd dress up, get in her truck, away we'd go to the St. Francis, dance half the night, compare notes after, while eating ham and eggs at Denny's. She always was the belle of the ball and had more boy friends than she could tuck away. On top of that, she decided she wanted to learn professional hair styling and went to beauty college along with all the bubble-headed teenagers. Got her license and opened her own shop."

In addition to sharing true-life stories, the mail brought good suggestions, some from people who had had ostomies, but more from people who had had other major surgery. They all warned me about the same thing— fatigue—and though I knew about that intellectually, I couldn't seem to remember it in practice. Any major surgery, especially abdominal surgery, slows one down. As I wrote to one of them: "Yes, impatience is the enemy. My surgery was two months ago yesterday and everyone, including the surgeon, thinks I'm getting along great, but there are times when I wonder. Part of my problem is feeling too good, relatively, so that about every other day I manage to overdo and then spend the next day catching up."

Phyllis had had a mastectomy and she said, "Be prepared to go into a wingding every time you feel an odd twinge. We become cowards and die a thousand deaths. First you're sure it's your brain (that's an easy one) or what was that sudden pain under the rib? You coughed! MY GOD. So if you can swing with all those little devils of metastasis, you've really got it made—but do get plenty of rest."

Even with that big headline, "A Colostomy," on my newspaper column, people could still wish me well—and ignore the details. "You're up and around?" "Oh yes. I had a bit of abdominal surgery and now I'm feeling better every day." "Good."

There's a lot of trial and error along the way, but walking gets easier, as do eating and staying up really late (like until ten o'clock!).

Part of the trick is that the energy to move comes from moving; on the other hand, the longer one stays in bed, the longer one stays in bed. It may take a month or two for even the most proper digestive system to get back to normal. A lot of the problems are in the head. If you think you're sick, it's harder to get well than if you think you're getting well (and after all, you survived spareribs and sauerkraut last night, so maybe it's true).

Some anonymous UOA member wrote, "Learning to live with the new ostomy may be a satisfactory adjustment, but it is not the best. It is better to decide that it is going to have to live with you in the kind of life you want to live. Surprisingly, if you truly mean it, the ostomy will be quite co-operative. The best adjustment I have seen is the patient who said quite sincerely, 'If God had stopped to think a bit, He would have put them on the abdomen to begin with.'"

If a parent of a young child has an ostomy, the most important part of the explanation is the reassurance that now Mom or Dad will be healthier. When a parent is ill or hospitalized, children often are terrified; they need to know that they are not in any way to blame. The physical explanations can be very simple. An ostomy is just a different place for the bowel movement or urine to come out of the body. This was necessary to make the parent healthy again.

Children are curious and may want to see pouches or the stoma. Parents can respond in whatever way they feel comfortable. In any case, openness and matter-of-factness are the best approaches. Children frequently surprise us with the maturity and caring of their responses.

Children's questions can't be shrugged off or avoided. My grandchildren were beyond the toddler stage, so Kerry took over the questions and answers before I got home from the hospital.

"Were they curious?" I asked the other day, years after the event.

"They still are—curious and quite supportive."

"How so?"

"Well, like Steve offered to do the drawings for *The Ostomy Book*. I told him two co-authors from one family were enough!"

CHAPTER 9 ❊ *Permanent*
Colostomies:
Changes and Choices

People have one thing in common;
they are all different.
Robert Zend

Colostomies have been around for a long time. The first ones, pretty much trial and error, were done about the time of the American Revolution and shortly thereafter. Nineteenth century medical journals bristled with debates about how, why, when, and where such surgery—first called a *preternatural anus* and later an *artificial anus*— should be performed. For a time, lumbar colostomies were favored, although it's hard to imagine how anyone managed a stoma located on the lower back. Since, with some exceptions, the patient's life expectancy wasn't very promising at that time, perhaps no one worried much about how to take care of the colostomy.

By the latter part of the 19th century, colostomies were becoming more common, but there were still monumental difficulties, both in doing the surgery and in surviving it. And yet, the body has such a strong will to survive, it often does, against very long odds. In 1968, the *Ostomy Quarterly* had a feature about Miss Miriam Coney, who underwent her colostomy surgery in 1884 at the age of 20. She survived eight brothers and sisters to celebrate 84 years with a colostomy *and* her 104th birthday in 1968!

The year 1908 was a turning point, when William Ernest Miles, M.D., performed the first *abdominoperineal (A-P) resection* of the rectum, still the standard surgery for many rectal cancers located close to the anal opening. The operation gets its name from the two incisions the surgeon makes: one through the abdomen and one through the perineum (the area between the genitals and the anus).

Through the abdominal incision, the surgeon cuts free from the surrounding tissue as much of the diseased part of the bowel as can be reached through this incision. A separate opening is cut on the abdomen for the future stoma. Finally the bowel is clamped and severed, with the healthy near end brought through the stoma opening, and the far end with the tumor temporarily left where it is.

Through the perineal incision, the surgeon frees the anus and rectum (and adjoining tissues, as needed), and then removes the whole diseased section of intestine. Since the body must have a constantly available exit for waste after food has been digested, removing the rectum and anus makes a colostomy necessary.

It's the location of the cancer which often determines whether a colostomy is necessary. If possible, the surgeon simply *resects* (cuts out) the tumor and *anastomoses* (joins) the two remaining healthy ends of intestine to function as before, with no colostomy. To anastamose the two ends, however, after the cancer and a safe swath of tissue around it have been removed, there has to be enough intestine left at the anal end to reconnect—and the anal sphincter muscles must be intact.

Sometimes the cancer occurs so near the end of the digestive tract that there just isn't an alternative to a colostomy and removal of the rectum and anus if the whole cancer is to be removed. It doesn't make sense for a surgeon to remove too little tissue and jeopardize the patient's chances of cure just to avoid a colostomy.

Until quite recently, many colostomies became necessary because, although there was enough healthy tissue at the anal end to reconnect, the surgeon couldn't reach it through the narrow bony vault which encloses the end of the digestive tract. Now, newer techniques and equipment (such as an ingenious surgical staple gun inserted through the anus which joins the two ends of intestine) have extended the surgeon's reach. This means fewer colostomies. (Also, some cancers, when small and just on the surface layer of the intestine, can be destroyed by radiation therapy.) If the rectum and anus must be removed, however, the colostomy is permanent.

Sometimes a colostomy is temporary, to divert feces away from an injury, diseased area, or a fresh surgical site in the lower digestive tract while it heals. The rectum and anus are left alone. (*Chapter 14* deals with the different kinds of temporary ostomies.)

The lower end of the digestive tract—colon, rectum, and anus—is shaped like a squatty question mark. This muscular tube, some six feet (two meters) long, has two main functions. The right side of the colon absorbs a great deal of water (and the minerals dissolved therein) from newly digested food. The middle and the left side of the colon transport and store residue until a convenient time and place for its disposal. No digestion takes place in the colon.

As food waste enters the colon from the ileum, the last segment of the small intestine, it is generally quite soft, even liquid. However, as this fecal matter makes its clockwise journey up the ascending colon, across the transverse colon, and down the descending and sigmoid colon to the rectum and anus, it becomes firmer as additional water is absorbed from the feces. (In spite of appearance, even firmer, "formed" stool is still 3/4 water and 1/4 solid material: undigested roughage, bacteria, some inorganic matter and a little protein. The typical brown color comes from bile.)

With the removal of the rectum and anus, and perhaps the end of the colon, what remains is the small intestine and most of the large intestine. Digestion of food and absorption of water and salts do not change at all.

What *is* lost is part of the gut's storage area—and the anus, with its sphincters (rings of muscle) which make voluntary control of bowel movements possible. With no more voluntary control, the person with a colostomy chooses and learns new techniques to manage the bowel. Regulating the bowels in a way that's personally acceptable is the secret of living comfortably with a colostomy.

The usual colostomy which results from an A-P resection is a *sigmoid colostomy*, so named because it is the healthy end of the sigmoid colon which is brought through the abdominal wall to form a stoma, after the rectum and anus are removed. Since the stool at this end of the digestive tract is fairly solid, the person with a sigmoid colostomy has some choices in how to cope with the ostomy: irrigation (basically, an enema through the stoma, done at a regular time every day or two); regulation by diet; or laissez-faire.

For years, in the United States, most health professionals urged everyone with a sigmoid colostomy to irrigate. Not to do so was considered not only to be courting a health disaster, but also somehow antisocial—almost immoral! But irrigation doesn't work for everyone (particularly those with an irritable bowel or with diarrhea for any reason), and some people just don't like it. In almost all cases, the bowel continues to function and pass stool quite nicely, with or without irrigation.

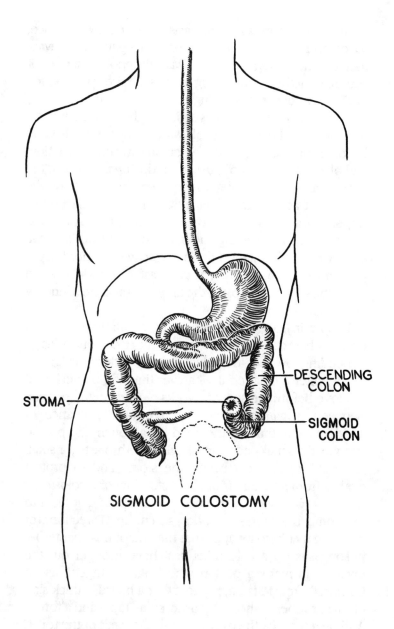

STOMA

DESCENDING COLON

SIGMOID COLON

SIGMOID COLOSTOMY

Now there's greater emphasis on one's own choice, based on personal preference, previous patterns of evacuation, and living situation. Many pepole change or combine methods (switching to laissez-faire and a pouch during a wilderness camping trip, for instance).

With irrigation, the bowel is taught to respond on schedule to the stimulus of water. The unpredictable becomes predictable, and the person can choose the time and place for evacuation. Irrigation does *not* wash out the bowel, and has nothing to do with the health of the intestinal tract. What it does is stretch the last section of digestive tract before the stoma; the intestine responds to this stimulus by pushing the irrigating fluid out and the stool with it. If irrigation done correctly does not keep a person free from stooling for at least 24 hours between irrigations—at least most of the time—it's a waste of energy and time.

People irrigate at the same time regularly every day, every other day (or even every third or fourth day), depending on the individual bowel pattern. Irrigating shortly after a meal or at whatever time the bowels used to move before the surgery works well for many people. Between irrigations, relatively free of the chance of accidents and, thus, of the need for a pouch, the person can wear a small pad, often backed with plastic; a small "security" pouch to cushion the stoma and to protect clothes from any mucus or slight stooling; or a colostomy "plug," a two-piece device with a foam plug that fits into the stoma, blocking stool, odor, and noise. (Directions for irrigating a colostomy appear at the end of this chapter.)

Long sits on a cold toilet seat have brought out the inventor in many a person who irrigates. Ingenious Ed Gambrell, from Atlanta, put together a board, a thick slab of foam rubber, a sheet of plastic, some tape, and a towel. Adding a terry cloth cover to warm the back of the toilet, he came up with his own "colostothrone," a comfortable skinny seat which fits on the back of the toilet seat. Cutting a U-shaped hole at the front bottom of a large sweat shirt, he had a "colostojacket" to keep him cosy no matter how icy the temperature. Many people use a foot-stool, and padded toilet seats are sold everywhere. Since relaxation is essential for a successful irrigation, it's worth looking around to see how physical and mental comfort can be increased (a hot drink, radio or TV, or a good book, maybe?).

In some households, privacy is a luxury, especially if there are others banging on the bathroom door. If a change in irrigation time doesn't work, compromise is in order. Ed Gambrell insists on privacy when he watches a ball game on TV while he irrigates. Otherwise, he resigns himself to a partial "open door policy." The kids can ask their questions. Everyone's happy.

Some bowels never adjust to irrigation. Other people just don't like the whole idea, or prefer to use their time differently. If bowel movements were regular before surgery, some people, with a little judicious attention to diet, may be able to encourage a tendency toward regularity again. Sometimes, juggling low-fiber foods, which tend to be constipating, with high and medium bulk foods can alter the consistency of the discharge, and may make the timing more predictable. This sort of regulation doesn't work when the stool is loose and frequent. During this early stage, the person wears a pouch all the time. Later, a pattern may emerge; perhaps more and more regularly, the bowels move after breakfast.

When the bowels move at an unexpected time, keeping track of the foods eaten in the previous two or three days, can give an idea of what foods to eat or avoid. While some people seem to be able to eat anything, others find they get diarrhea or excessive gas from very spicy foods, foods high in elemental sulphur and iron (onions, cabbage), or other particular kinds of food. (Often people who have trouble with one kind of food at some point can tolerate it later.) Once the colostomy learns to behave docilely, in response to food, a few people can attach an appliance when the bowel movement is expected, and wear a light covering over the stoma at other times. Most still wear a pouch all the time, however. The records are skimpy, but complete control by diet appears to be rare. Drugs which slow the bowel are added sometimes, but they have their own hazards. Further experimentation might develop more dependable approaches.

Then there is the laissez-faire approach. This involves wearing a drainable pouch all the time, emptying it when necessary, and otherwise letting the colon go its own way. (A colostomy "plug" is an option for periods of a few hours—for swimming, perhaps, or sexual relations.) Some colostomies never respond to irrigation or diet control, and some people just prefer this simple method of management. This method does mean the expense of pouches, however.

Since most fecal matter from sigmoid colostomies is fairly solid, and thus doesn't pool on the skin, most people aren't plagued with major skin problems. Cleaning gently but thoroughly around the stoma, changing pouches regularly, and keeping away from products which cause allergic skin reactions help maintain healthy skin around the stoma.

Just about everyone with a colostomy suffers occasionally from diarrhea or looseness of stool—from that 24-hour flu bug, an antibiotic, those extra-spicy enchiladas, or as a side effect of radiation therapy. Time, a change in diet, and perhaps anti-diarrhea medication usually take care of it. Irrigation should be postponed until the bowel slows down again. This is the time to dig out that emergency drainable pouch.

Constipation (hardness of stool) may be a problem. If the problem continues, it may help to add more high-fiber foods to the diet: bran, fruit and vegetables, whole grain breads, for instance. Some of the bulk-producing laxatives, taken with plenty of fluids, can work as stool softeners. (Irritating laxatives can cause trouble if taken more than occasionally.) More fluids, regular exercise, a cup of hot liquid, a soothing bath, any relaxing activity, are home remedies for constipation. Narcotic pain medications are notorious constipation-causers, as are iron pills and antihistamines. If these are factors, the doctor may be able to suggest a change in medication. In any case, if the problem lasts for a while, it's definitely time to visit the doctor.

For everyone with a colostomy, managing this new change in the plumbing is a challenge. Fred E. Bradford, MD, sums it up: "Learning to manage a colostomy is much simpler than learning to ride a bicycle, and no one ever mastered the bike who quit after the first fall."

IRRIGATING A COLOSTOMY

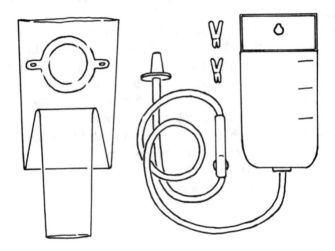

1. Like a regular enema bag and tubing, an irrigation kit contains
a bag for the irrigation fluid, usually water. This bag is attached
to a tube which has a clamp to adjust water flow. Many people
with colostomies prefer to use a soft plastic cone at the end
of the tube. Effective and safe, this cone fits snugly against
the stoma, keeps fluid from returning until it is supposed to,
and prevents any chance of damage to the intestinal lining.

   An irrigating sleeve attaches over the stoma and is long
enough to reach into the toilet bowl. The sleeve is open at
both the top (for access to the stoma) and the bottom (for
discharge of stool and water into the toilet).

   Also in the irrigation kit are clips to close the irrigating
sleeve after the irrigation process is partially complete.

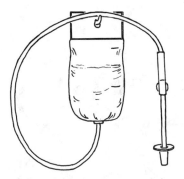

2. With the water-flow clamp on the tube closed, fill the irrigation bag with about two to four measuring cups lukewarm water, and hang the bag on a sturdy hook; the bottom of the bag will be at shoulder height when you are sitting. Release the water-flow clamp slowly so that water runs through the tube to clear out any air. The clamp is closed again.

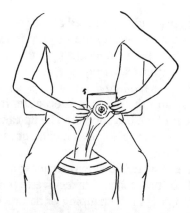

3. You can sit on the toilet or on a chair facing the toilet. The irrigating sleeve is placed over the stoma and snapped on and/or held in place with a belt. The bottom end of the sleeve rests in the toilet above the water. The end can be cut or cuffed, if necessary.

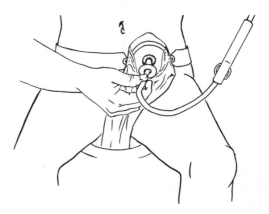

4. The cone is lubricated with a non-greasy medical lubricant jelly (not petroleum jelly), brought through the open top of the irrigating sleeve, and held in place firmly against the stoma.

    If you use an irrigating tip instead of the cone, the distance the tip is to be inserted into the ostomy is measured and marked on the tube beforehand; the tip is then lubricated and inserted into the stoma with a gentle, rolling motion. A dam (a flat, doughnut-shaped device that encircles the irrigating tube) is held against the stoma to keep water from escaping around the sides of the irrigation tip. The tip carries more risk of perforating the intestine than the cone does and must be used very carefully.

5. Open the water-flow clamp slowly to allow a gentle stream of water to enter the stoma; it takes five to ten minutes for all the water to flow in. If cramping or nausea occur during this period, the usual culprit is too much water, water that is too cold or hot, or too fast a flow. Some people find that if they wait five minutes or so more after the water flows in before removing the cone or irrigating tip, they get a more complete irrigation.

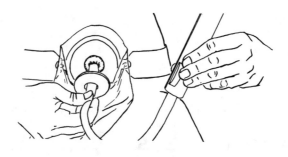

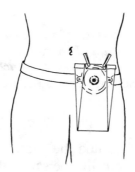

6. Remove the cone or irrigating tip from the stoma. Most of the irrigation returns come in spurts into the toilet during the first 10 to 15 minutes. After this period, you can use the clips to close the open ends of the irrigating sleeve and can attend to other business. Some find that gentle massage along the path of the colon, a hot drink, deep breathing, or mild exercise speeds up the return of stool during the next half hour or so. Before long, you will learn how it feels when all the water and bowel movement have been expelled. Then the irrigating sleeve is removed. Many people enjoy a shower or bath before applying a soft pad or security pouch over the stoma, and cleaning the irrigation equipment. Washing the irrigating sleeve with cool water keeps odors from being sealed in.

CHAPTER 10

❧ *Ileostomies and Alternatives*

> *So much of my life has been devoted to an ulcerated colon which no longer exists. . .such a waste of time.*
> Norbert Hertel, speaking of his ileostomy

If you ever need to find the nearest bathroom in a strange town, seek out the person with inflammatory bowel disease. Along with his mental map of every bathroom in town, he can probably tell you about the local hospitals: He's been in them enough.

But, no matter how much the disease has disrupted his life, when the typical person with inflammatory bowel disease hears about the hope an ileostomy may offer, he balks. So may his family and even his doctor. If it becomes a life-or-death choice, he still despairs: "An ostomy? How can I live with something. . .like that?"

After surgery and recovery, he asks a different question: "Why did I *ever* wait so long?"

Although there's no such thing as a *typical* person with an ostomy, those who have had ileostomies share some striking similarities. Most are young and undergo surgery after devastating sieges of inflammatory bowel disease. And most, after recovering from surgery, resume life— whether school, career, raising a family or whatever—with abundant energy and enthusiasm.

Such happy endings are relatively new.

Inflammatory bowel diseases have been around for a long time. Bonnie Prince Charlie supposedly suffered from one, as did Beethoven. Roman Emperor Claudius had the symptoms of "the bloody flux" and, as Dr. F. T. de Domnal reports, a physician from Ephesus (named, incredibly, Soranus!) wrote a quite adequate description of inflammatory bowel disease in 117 A.D.

Inflammatory bowel disease (IBD) is the term for two diseases which attack the intestinal tract. Both *ulcerative colitis* and *Crohn's disease* are chronic diseases which come and go unpredictably. The symptoms—such as persistent diarrhea (often with blood and/or mucus), abdominal pain or cramps, fever and weight loss, and (sometimes) joint pains and/or skin or eye irritations— come from the immune system's inflammatory response to some "enemy." However, instead of the bowel's normal inflammatory response of flushing an offending agent out of the body with diarrhea and then quieting, the inflammatory response in IBD keeps escalating, building on itself, causing more damage than any "enemy" could. Sometimes IBD can be relatively mild, with an occasional bothersome attack, but it can also be a debilitating, life-threatening disease.

Ulcerative colitis batters the colon and rectum, destroying the mucous lining of the large intestine in bouts of severe, often bloody, diarrhea. The colitis flares and recedes, usually starting in the rectum and progressing methodically upward through the colon, from one area to the adjoining one. If the colon and the mucous lining of the rectum are removed, the disease is gone forever.

Crohn's disease (named after the New York physician

who described it in 1932) can involve all the layers of the bowel. It can occur anywhere in the digestive tract from the mouth to the anus, but it most often targets the last section of the small intestine, the terminal ileum. Other common names for Crohn's disease include *ileitis* (when it involves mostly the ileum), *regional enteritis* (from the Greek work *enteron*, meaning "intestine"), *Crohn's colitis* (when only the colon seems to be affected), or *granulomatous disease of the bowel* (from the appearance of the diseased intestine under a microscope).

Crohn's disease tends to "skip around" the bowel, with diseased areas sandwiching sections of normal bowel. Crohn's can also cause such problems as *fistulas* (abnormal tunnelings from one body organ to another), and abscesses around the anus. The disease may disappear, if the terminal ileum and the colon are removed, but it can also come back elsewhere in the digestive tract; thus, surgery is said to bring about a *remission* (which may or may not be permanent) rather than a cure.

Doctors diagnose about 30,000 new cases of IBD in North America each year. They use barium x-ray studies to show the contours of the whole digestive tract, and look directly at as much of the tract as they can see through the *endoscope* and/or colonoscope (tubes inserted through the mouth to look at the upper digestive tract or through the anus to look at the lower). Pathology doctors examine biopsy specimens taken through the scopes.

Most of the time it's relatively easy for doctors to diagnose IBD and to tell whether the IBD is ulcerative colitis or Crohn's disease, but not always. It's important to have a clear-cut diagnosis before some surgical procedures which cure ulcerative colitis but may cause more problems for the person with Crohn's.

IBD typically strikes teenagers and young adults, with a second smaller but sizable group of patients over 60. Many people with IBD have a relative with the disease.

The risk of colorectal cancer rises dramatically for people with ulcerative colitis for more than 10 to 20 years; people with Crohn's may face some increased risk.

What causes inflammatory bowel disease? No one knows yet. In 1966, what is now the Crohn's and Colitis Foundation of America, Inc., or CCFA (formerly the National Foundation for Ileitis and Colitis, Inc.) was formed to help find out why. CCFA raises money for research into causes and treatment, sponsors seminars and supplies literature to reach doctors and nurses, and provides information, support groups and hospital visitation programs for people with IBD.

Researchers have learned that neither diet nor stress causes IBD (although either can make an existing case worse). Scientists are looking at such factors as heredity, certain kinds of infectious agents, and immune system abnormalities.

Meanwhile, medicines which reduce inflammation (such as steroids and salicylate drugs) can ease the symptoms of inflammatory bowel disease, although they cannot cure it. Other medicines for IBD include antibiotics and drugs for pain and diarrhea.

In some cases, doctors may use medicines which suppress the immune system, the same powerful drugs that patients use to keep their bodies from rejecting a transplanted kidney, liver, or heart. The theory is that IBD may happen because the body, for some reason, begins to see its own bowel as an enemy, as not belonging to itself, and tries to "reject" it.

Getting adequate nutrition during flare-ups of IBD—when food may travel through the gut too quickly to be absorbed fully, and when eating anything can lead to abdominal cramping and diarrhea—can be challenging indeed. Some IBD patients can eat anything, any time. Others find that they have less diarrhea and abdominal cramping with a bland, low-fiber diet (avoiding fruits, vegetables, raisins, nuts, seeds, and whole grains) when the disease is active. If areas of the small bowel become narrowed, as can happen with Crohn's disease, the patient chooses a minimal residue (low-fiber) diet or even a liquid diet to prevent total blockage. Like people without IBD who have an allergy to milk, many people with IBD cannot tolerate lactose, the sugar present in most milk products, and do much better when they cut dairy foods out of their diets.

Hospitalization is necessary if a patient becomes dehydrated or acutely malnourished from diarrhea, or severely anemic from blood loss. Intravenous fluids and blood transfusions are common therapies. In some cases, proteins and other nutrients are given through a vein: *total parenteral nutrition*, (TPN) through a large "central" vein or a less-concentrated solution called *peripheral parenteral nutrition* (PPN) through a smaller arm vein. This *hyperalimentation* (another name for TPN or PPN) nourishes the body while the intestines get a chance to rest.

For most patients, this supportive treatment works well. But some people's disease doesn't respond to these treatments. Others with long-term ulcerative colitis may start showing precancerous changes in the bowel. Surgery becomes the only practical option.

One other group of IBD patients seeks surgery: those with severe disease who need heavy, constant doses of drugs, and for whom the treatment becomes almost as bad as the disease. As artist Reba Dockterman recalls about the years before her ileostomy: "There was little dignity left in my life as poverty took over, only over-shadowed by pain.

"The years inched by. I was no longer a model, a job I'd enjoyed with pride before my illness gave me a bloated tummy and my drugs puffed my cheeks into a moon-shaped face. My skin was modulated between shades of red to violet, my fingernails were completely concave, and the dark circles under my eyes could not be covered by the heaviest of makeups."

Reba brought up the possibility of ostomy surgery to her doctor. Like some doctors, he hesitated, because, "I'd hate to do that to you unless I have to." Finally, however, after the many hospitalizations, weight loss, dehydration, constant pain, weakness, utter misery, bleeding, harrowing social consequences—all common experiences for those with severe inflammatory bowel disease—Reba had an ileostomy.

Until the last few years, she wouldn't have had that option. Back in 1730, a Mrs. Margaret White underwent ileostomy surgery after rupture of a hernia containing the end of her ileum. She survived, but was housebound for the rest of her life.

Then in 1913, Dr. John Young Brown in St. Louis constructed the first ileostomy in the U.S. At that point, and for many years to come, an ileostomy remained a real horror story. Patients became dehydrated and died. With a primitive arsenal of medicines, surgeons watched their patients die of infection. Those who survived had towels and pads and whatever they could improvise to contain drainage. One company made "appliances": bulky, rubber, poorly-fitted pouches.

But gradually the picture brightened. In the early 1950s, shortly after a functional, drainable ostomy pouch was invented, British surgeon Bryan Brooke devised an ileostomy which really worked—and which is still the standard conventional ileostomy. Constructing a stoma by folding the end of the ileum back on itself like the neck of a turtleneck sweater, he avoided the problems which had made ileostomy surgery "a living death": rampant infection inside the stoma right after surgery and, if one lived through that, later narrowing and obstruction of the stoma. Surgeon Rupert Turnbull, of the Cleveland Clinic, brought the Brooke procedure to the United States. Medical

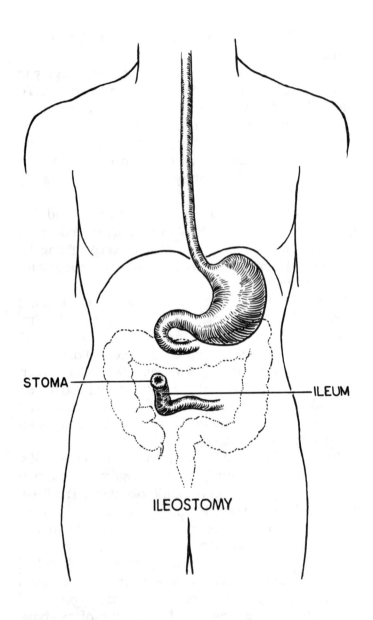

STOMA

ILEUM

ILEOSTOMY

Continent ileostomy with catheter in place

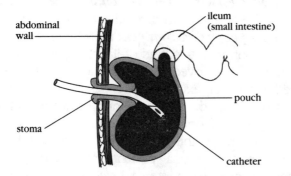

abdominal wall
ileum (small intestine)
pouch
stoma
catheter

advances such as antibiotics helped. At last, surgery could provide an almost instant cure for ulcerative colitis and often a permanent remission of Crohn's disease.

An ileostomy is a surgically-created opening through the abdominal wall so that body wastes can be expelled. The surgeon removes or bypasses the diseased colon (and in some cases of Crohn's disease, perhaps also a hefty section of the small intestine) and brings the remaining end of the ileum through the abdominal wall to form a stoma, usually on the lower right side of the abdomen. If the whole colon is removed, the surgery is called a *total colectomy*, (not to be confused with a colostomy, in which at least part of the colon remains in the body and is used to make the stoma). The removal of the rectum along with the whole colon is called a *total proctocolectomy* or *coloproctectomy*.

If, along with removing the entire colon, the surgeon takes out the whole rectum, there is no way to leave the anus, and a permanent ileostomy becomes necessary. The operation to remove the rectum and anus is called an *abdominoperineal resection* or A-P resection. (For a description of an A-P resection, see Chapter 9, page 74.) A plastic external pouch substitutes for the old storage area of colon and rectum.

In 1969, Swedish surgeon Nils Kock (pronounced like the cola beverage) introduced the *continent ileostomy,* an option for the patient with ulcerative colitis; this is also called a *Kock pouch* or a *continent intestinal reservoir* or CIR. The person with this kind of ileostomy has had the rectum and anus removed along with the colon, but does not need to wear an external pouch.

In this operation, the surgeon loops the last part of the ileum back on itself, opens the loop, and constructs from it a reservoir inside the abdomen. A narrow tube of intestine from this internal pouch tunnels through the abdomen to form a tiny stoma level with the skin. A one-way valve at the outlet of the reservoir keeps the stool from coming out—makes the ostomy "continent"— except when the person inserts a catheter a few times day to drain the reservoir (two or three times a day with a mature continent ileostomy). The reservoir stretches gradually until it holds a pint or more.

A fairly common problem with the continent ileostomy has been failure of the one-way valve so that the reservoir is no longer continent and/or it is difficult to insert the catheter. Modifications in the surgical techniques for making the one-way valve and the support for it have made valve failure much less likely, if the procedure is performed by a surgeon who does it frequently and uses these newer techniques.

The continent ileostomy procedure can be done as the first surgery for ulcerative colitis but often is used now as a conversion option for the person who already has a conventional Brooke ileostomy, and has had the rectum and anus removed. (For instance, the person who experiences major problems with the skin around the stoma of a conventional ileostomy may do very well with a continent ileostomy.)

Surgeons have another kind of internal reservoir to offer the person with ulcerative colitis who still has an

Ileoanal anastomosis with reservoir

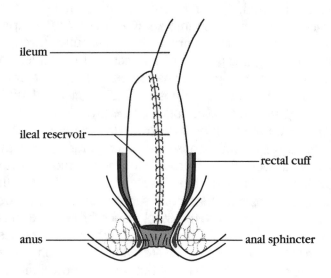

ileum

ileal reservoir

rectal cuff

anus

anal sphincter

intact, though diseased, digestive tract. This one, also made from a loop of the ileum, is then connected to the anus, so that stool will pass through the anal sphincters; no permanent ostomy is necessary.

The surgeon first removes the colon, the upper rectum, and just the surface layer of the last inch (2.5 cm) or so of the rectum. This eliminates both the ulcerative colitis, which attacks only the surface layer, and the risk of rectal cancer. However, lacking a colon and a storage area for stool, the person would have severe diarrhea and incontinence—were it not for the new internal storage area the surgeon makes.

To construct this reservoir, the surgeon loops the last section of the ileum, opens the intestine along the loop, and sews it in such a way as to create an *ileal reservoir* or pouch from the reconstructed "tubes." The surgeon can loop the ileum once, like the letter "J"; the resulting reservoir is called a "J" pouch and is the shape most commonly used. Larger reservoirs can be made if the surgeon loops the ileum into an "S" or even a "W" shape. When the reservoir is complete, its end is pulled through the remaining rectal "sleeve" and stitched or stapled to the anus; this joining is an anastomosis. (These surgeries are called by several names, including *ileoanal pull-through procedure, pelvic pouch procedure, ileoanal anastomosis with reservoir,* or *ileal pouch-anal anastomosis.*)

The surgeon often constructs a temporary ileostomy for several weeks or months to give the reservoir time to heal before it is used. (See Chapter 14 about living with a temporary ostomy.) A second surgery "takes down" the temporary ileostomy so that stool passes through the anus again. Within about six months, as the reservoir stretches and as the body adjusts to life without a colon, most patients find that they have about five soft bowel movements during the day and perhaps one at night. (Some continue to have problems with continence and with skin problems around the anus.)

Either the continent ileostomy or the ileoanal anastomosis reservoir can develop *pouchitis,* an inflammation which causes abdominal cramping pain, bloating, and a watery discharge. This can usually be treated successfully with antibiotics.

Neither a continent ileostomy nor an ileoanal anastomosis reservoir is recommended for the patient with Crohn's disease. The Crohn's tends to recur both in the reservoir, which then needs to be removed, and elsewhere in the digestive tract, leaving the person with less small intestine available for digestion. There is a high risk of developing *small bowel syndrome,* in which there is not enough intestine left to absorb the nutrients necessary for life.

With Crohn's disease, a surgical priority is preserving

as much as possible of the small intestine. With Crohn's colitis, the surgeon may be able to remove the colon and simply attach the end of the ileum to the upper end of the rectum. This is called an *ileorectal anastomosis* and saves the rectum and the anal sphincters so that stool passes through the anus as before, without a permanent ileostomy. (Often, the surgeon constructs a temporary ostomy for several weeks so the surgical connections can heal without stool passing over them.)

This surgery is also sometimes done for the ulcerative colitis patient with little or no apparent disease in the rectum. It leaves in place the rectum, still vulnerable to a recurrence of the disease, as well as to a significant risk of cancer; the rectum needs to be checked frequently.

If the anal sphincter is strong, and if the rectum stretches enough to act as an adequate storage area for the softer stool the body produces without a colon, continence may eventually become good. The person still passes several stools a day.

Besides IBD patients, there is another group of people who are potential candidates for either a conventional ileostomy or one of the alternative procedures: those with inherited diseases which cause hundreds, even thousands, of polyps in the large intestine. People with *familial polyposis* (also called familial polyposis coli or hereditary multiple polyposis) or *Gardner's Syndrome* face inevitable colorectal cancer in adulthood if the colon and (often) the rectum aren't removed. If the rectum is involved, a conventional ileostomy or one of the internal reservoirs is appropriate. If the rectum does not have multiple polyps, an ileorectal anastamosis, removing only the colon, is an option; the rectum then needs to be checked regularly.

Whatever the reason for the surgery, the person needs plenty of physical and emotional support. If possible, surgeons try to perform surgery on IBD patients when the disease is relatively quiet; some may need building up before surgery, perhaps through intravenous fluids and total parenteral nutrition. Medication may need to be changed, especially if the patient has been taking high doses of steroids, which would slow wound healing.

In retrospect, those first few days after an ileostomy seem unreal. Jane Walker, an ET from Atlanta, Georgia, writes: "It is difficult, many times, for us to remember what it is like to be a new ileostomate. Looking back, do you remember the first feelings of something 'alive' on your abdomen as you experienced the peristaltic action of the stoma? How about the feeling of warm stool draining into the disposable pouch, wondering if it was 'in or out' of the pouch and looking to see? Did you carry a sack full of supplies everywhere you went, afraid you would break a seal? Do you remember, in your early post-op days, holding your hand on your pouch or stoma when you walked. Don't kid yourself, you did too, and probably still do at times."

But those first days pass quickly. One day the person with the new ileostomy realizes he or she has gone *thirty minutes* without even being aware of the ostomy! Confidence builds as one masters techniques for emptying and applying pouches, or for using a catheter if there is a continent ileostomy. Before long, such chores are just part of the daily routine, along with brushing one's teeth.

The person with an ileostomy may have concerns about odor (see *Chapter 12—Pouches and the Skin They Touch*) and gas (*Chapter 15—Eating Well*). If the rectum and anus have been removed, there will be a perineal wound which may be tender for a time (*Chapter 6—On the Mend*). Food *blockage* which obstructs the small intestine, and, for those who have had a large portion of the small intestine removed, vitamin B_{12} absorption may become problems (see *Chapter 15—Eating Well*).

But people with ileostomies, whether permanent or

temporary, have some special challenges, some from the loss of the colon and some from the nature of body waste when it reaches the stoma. The body usually functions quite nicely without the colon and rectum, but has lost some of its ability to absorb water, salt and potassium. With a new ileostomy, waste will still be quite liquid when it reaches the stoma. Eventually, the small intestine may compensate somewhat for the loss of the colon, and the stool may become thicker, perhaps pasty in consistency. The kidneys continue to adjust the water balance and the urine may become more concentrated as the body loses water in the stool. Drinking *lots* of fluids does *not* make the feces more liquid, and *does* help the kidneys wash out the chemicals which can lead to gallstones or kidney stones, potential hazards after years with an ileostomy. Especially during hot weather or hard physical activity, the person without a colon needs to keep an eye on replenishing water, salt, and potassium.

Until the digestive tract starts functioning again after surgery (usually a few days), there's no stool. When peristalsis finally returns, the ostomy is often on its *worst* behavior. Stool may be constant and watery.

Time tames many ileostomies. But it's an individual matter. Some people can set a clock by their stomas: Half an hour after they eat, "Vesuvius" erupts. Others, including many of those who have had some of the small intestine removed at the same time, continue to have more frequent discharge. For many, there are predictable times of peace, especially during the morning hours.

The small intestine's specialty is digesting food, breaking it up into tiny pieces with the help of enzymes. Given a chance, those same intestinal enzymes which will digest a New York steak will do the same thing to any skin they touch.

When fashioning the ileostomy, the surgeon ideally creates a stoma which extends 3/4 to one inch (about 2 cm) beyond the abdomen. Thus, the ileum discharges directly into the pouch and away from the skin. But it still takes special care to protect the skin around the stoma and to keep the pouch seal secure. Cleaning the area well but gently, using ostomy products to which the skin is tolerant, watching for any break in the seal which means a pouch change is necessary all contribute to healthy skin.

Timed-release and other coated medicine capsules and pills which are supposed to be absorbed in the colon, may pass whole through an ileostomy. Many medicines are available in liquid form; some others can be removed from capsules. The doctor or pharmacist can advise. The person with the ileostomy should remind the doctor or pharmacist to provide medication in the right form.

Mae West said it: "When choosing between two evils, I always like to try the one I've never tried before."

An ileostomy's no evil—as thousands of people who have them can attest—although it's certainly new and strange and unfamiliar at first. But when one remembers what the ileostomy replaces. . .

As Michele says, "Anyone who wants the battered, tortured intestine I got rid of, is more than welcome to it! I don't hurt any more. I can eat. I can work. Sure, sometimes it's a bother—but I love my ileostomy.

"I can *live* now!"

CHAPTER 11 ❈ *Life Without a Built-in Bladder*

*The urinary stoma is the only stoma
that is connected directly to a life
supporting system—the kidneys.*
Katherine F. Jeter, ET

People who have a urostomy, a surgical opening in the abdominal wall so that urine is diverted away from a diseased or defective part of the urinary tract, come in all different sizes and ages. Baby Steve, cooing and drooling like any five-month-old, is a veteran already because he was born with a serious urinary tract defect. Six-year-old Patti Anne treasures her new ruffled panties—a urostomy spells freedom from constant diapers and "Baby, Baby, Patti!" taunts from her playmates; a spinal defect meant that she couldn't control urination before her surgery.

Jim, 22, needed a temporary urostomy until he grew strong enough to withstand major repair of car accident injuries to his urinary tract. To 55-year-old Tom, a urostomy means he has exchanged a cancerous bladder for an external pouch, and a new lease on life. For Susan, 48, a urostomy and a colostomy were part of the massive surgery necessary to give her a chance at life after cancer of the cervix spread through her pelvis.

Whatever the difference in their immediate reasons for surgery, Steve, Patti Anne, Jim, Tom and Susan (and thousands of others like them) all underwent urostomy surgery to provide a safe and reliable passageway out of the body for urine.

Twenty-four hours a day, a veritable Niagara of blood rushes through the two kidneys, small but essential organs, one on each side of the spinal column. Each minute, an adult male's kidneys filter about five cups of blood through two million nephrons, tiny processing stations which flush waste and then return the purified blood to the circulatory system. Responding to hormones, the kidneys also maintain the balance of water and other substances like sodium and potassium in the body.

Each kidney empties urine it has made into a ureter, a narrow, muscular tube which propels the fluid, with a milking action, through a special one-way valve into the bladder. The bladder is basically a reservoir, supplied with muscle and nerves, to hold urine until it is convenient to dispose of it. From the bladder, urine travels through the urethra, a simple passageway to the outside. The nerve supply to the urethra makes it open and close at the right times.

This whole system is a sterile one: Urine leaving the body should be completely free of bacteria. Even if infection reaches the bladder through the urethra, ordinarily the one-way valve on each ureter protects the kidneys.

At least some kidney function, and some means of removing the urine from the body, are essential for life. Any condition which seriously interrupts the flow of urine to the outside can lead to an ostomy. All urostomies are urinary diversions, done to reroute the urinary tract, although not all urinary diversions result in stomas. Where it occurs in the urinary tract and how the surgery is done give the particular ostomy its name.

Some surgeries are relatively easy and straightforward to do, and are performed primarily for patients who are too weak and ill for more difficult surgery. They are also useful stopgap procedures for very young patients who need to grow bigger before they have corrective surgeries.

In one type of urinary diversion, a *nephrostomy* (from the Greek word for "kidney"), a plastic tube is inserted through the skin directly into the kidney; the tube stays in place, draining urine, as long as it's needed. If the problem occurs farther down in the urinary tract, the surgeon can bring one or both ureters through the abdominal wall during *ureterostomy* surgery. In other procedures, the bladder can open on the abdominal wall directly or by way of a plastic tube with a *vesicostomy* or a *cystostomy* (both from Greek words for "bladder").

Relatively simple operations these may be, and lifesaving in many cases, but they present so many difficulties after surgery that they usually are not considered as permanent solutions for urinary tract problems. When it is brought to the surface of the body, the narrow ureter tends to scar and close off. The vesicostomy, because of its location in the pubic area, can be quite difficult to manage; pubic hair and the shape of the lower pelvis make pouches hard to attach and maintain. And the closer the ostomy is to the kidney, the smaller is the margin of safety for protecting the kidney from infection.

With these kinds of urinary diversions, the surgeon bypasses the bladder but usually does not remove it. If the underlying problem is corrected later, the urinary diversion can be reversed (*undiversion*). This happens commonly in children who grow big enough for urinary tract reconstruction surgeries.

If the bladder is removed (*total cystectomy*), the urostomy is considered permanent. People who need a total cystectomy and can tolerate major surgery usually undergo an operation in which a segment of intestine is fashioned into a conduit, or passageway, for urine to the outside.

Dr. Bricker gets credit for developing, in the 1940s and 50s, what remains the most common permanent urostomy, the *ileal conduit*, also known as a Bricker or ileal loop. Although the surgery is complicated, the idea is simple. The surgeon cuts a short section of the ileum away from the rest of the small intestine. This detached segment can then be moved, along with its nerve and blood supply, so that ureters can be attached to it. The surgeon closes one end of the segment and brings the other end through the abdominal wall to form a stoma. (The two ends of the remaining small intestine are reconnected, so that bowel movements pass as they did before.)

The ileal conduit is not to be confused with an ileostomy, which is for stool. Despite the fact that a piece of intestine is used in the construction of the ileal conduit, the urostomy passes only urine.

The detached segment of the ileum serves as a passageway for urine to the outside. Since the nerve and blood supplies remain, the segment continues peristalsis, the normal intestinal pulsation which keeps the urine moving away from the kidneys. Since an ileal conduit is not a bladder, one needs an external pouch, securely fastened to the skin, to act as a bladder; the emptying spout of the pouch takes the place of the urethra. The normal kidneys produce several drops of urine each minute around the clock, so drainage is constant.

The ileal conduit is still far from a perfect solution (although it works remarkably well). The one-way valve from ureter to bladder is missing, so the kidneys have limited protection from urine backflow and possible infection. In fact, infection is quite rare; if it occurs, it usually responds readily to antibiotics.

Sometimes surgeons use a piece of the colon rather

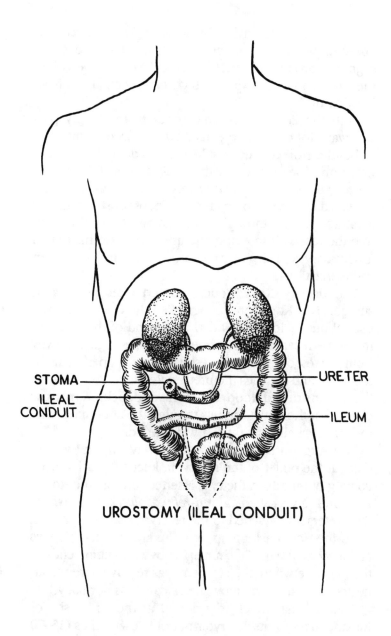

STOMA

ILEAL
CONDUIT

URETER

ILEUM

UROSTOMY (ILEAL CONDUIT)

than the ileum to make the conduit, called a *colonic conduit.* When the ureters are attached to the colon segment through a tunnel between layers of the colon, the tunnel makes a valve which may keep urine from backing up into the kidneys.

Both the ileal and colonic conduits are simply passageways for urine. Surgeons now are developing ways to build a storage area, a substitute bladder. A continent urostomy, for instance—either a Kock pouch or an *Indiana pouch*—is an internal reservoir for urine. A few times a day, the person with a continent urostomy inserts a catheter (tube) through a tiny stoma on the abdomen into the reservoir to empty the urine. No external pouch is necessary; a small gauze pad protects the stoma between catheterizations.

The urinary Kock pouch, named after its creator, surgeon Nils Kock (pronounced like the cola beverage), uses about 12 inches (30 cm) at the end of the ileum to make the reservoir. The surgeon cuts this segment away from the rest of the small intestine, loops it, opens it along the loop, and attaches the ureters. Refolded and stitched, the reconstructed loop becomes a pouch. A narrow channel at the outlet tunnels through the abdominal wall to form a small stoma, flush with the skin.

The surgeon constructs two one-way "nipple" valves. One, at the outlet of the reservoir, keeps the urine from coming out until a catheter is inserted through the stoma. A second valve, called an *anti-reflux valve,* is made where the ureters are attached to the reservoir; it helps prevent the urine from backing up, or refluxing, into the kidneys and injuring them. (Of course, the two remaining ends of the intestine where the segment was removed are reconnected so that bowel movements can pass normally.)

The Indiana pouch, developed at the University of Indiana, uses for its reservoir not only 6–8 inches (15–20 cm) at the end of the ileum, but also the cecum and ascending colon at the beginning of the large intestine. The segment of large intestine, detached from the intestinal tract is opened, and the ureters are sewn in place, using an anti-reflux technique, so that urine won't back up into the kidneys. The surgeon then folds the opened bowel and closes it to form a spherical reservoir. The piece of ileum, still connected to the reservoir, is "pleated" to make it smaller in diameter and then is brought through the abdominal wall to form a tiny flush stoma.

In another recently-developed procedure, some surgeons construct an internal reservoir (similar to the reservoir in a continent urostomy), as a substitute bladder, and connect it directly to the urethra, so that urine exits the body through the urethra. This means no stoma and no need to drain urine through a catheter. However, this operation is available now only for men, because it requires the longer urethra that men have.

A new option for women combines a small pouch, like that from a continent urostomy, attached internally to the rectum. This reservoir provides some storage for urine, which then exits the body along with stool through the anus. The valves in the reservoir help protect the kidneys from urine backflow and from the bacteria in the rectum.

These bladder substitute procedures have their own risks and complications. New refinements keep appearing to make them safer, more effective surgeries, but they continue to be measured against the ileal conduit, still the "gold standard" operation.

Recent developments in the treatment of early bladder cancers mean that sometimes the bladder can be saved and no urostomy is needed. Such therapies include minor surgery which removes only the cancer and preserves the urinary tract, chemotherapy (sometimes with drugs applied directly to the bladder), and assorted radiation therapy techniques.

There are other options now for people with severe

urinary incontinence (the inability to hold urine) who used to have few choices except diapers and urostomy surgeries. Now, many use *intermittent catheterization*, in which the person or a family member drains the bladder a few times a day with a catheter. Surgeons are also experimenting with an artificial urinary sphincter to control the passage of urine out of the body. A bladder pacemaker, an electronic device which signals when the bladder needs emptying, is a possibility for those with damage to the nerves which control urination. (Help for Incontinent People, or HIP, provides information about current and upcoming treatments through a periodic newsletter and brochures: P.O. Box 544, Union, SC 29379.)

Before any urinary diversion surgery, patients undergo such tests as standard x-rays of the whole urinary tract, and *intravenous pyelograms* (IVPs), special x-rays taken after medicine is injected through an arm vein and travels through the urinary tract. The doctor also looks directly into the bladder through a *cystoscope*, a lighted tube inserted through the urethra. Any urinary diversion which uses a piece of intestine means that a full "bowel prep," complete with laxatives and/or enemas plus antibiotics is necessary before surgery. This reduces the chance of infection after surgery.

Those first days after surgery can be a bit harrowing. Along with the incision and the stoma, red and moist, there are tubes and drains. These may include *stents*, narrow plastic tubes threaded through each ureter from the conduit to protect the ureter-conduit connections while they heal; these stents protrude from the stoma and are removed after a few days. (Removing stents is not painful.)

The pouch, frequently from a limited hospital stock, will be hooked up to a bedside receptacle all the time at first. Eventually, the patient with the new urostomy learns to empty the pouch regularly; then it is connected to the bedside receptacle only at night. It may take some time—and trial and error—to find the best, most comfortable and workable pouch.

With the deluge of information in the weeks after urostomy surgery, it seems difficult at first to separate the crucial from the less important. It is not as complicated as it may appear.

The *most* important consideration for anyone with a urostomy is to keep the kidneys functioning smoothly; this must be a real *commitment*. In most urostomies done now, the kidneys empty, after a brief passage with no one-way valves, into an outside pouch. This means less protection from infection, more chance of urine backing up into the kidneys with a load of bacteria. Fortunately, in most cases, with good care, no problem develops.

But preventing kidney infection involves some common-sense measures. If the urine flows well, and stays away from the stoma, infection is rare. This means checking fairly often that urine continues to flow. One hour without urine in the pouch is too long: Medical help is necessary. Bacteria multiply rapidly in urine. This means using *clean* pouches, either disposable ones, or else reusable ones, thoroughly scrubbed and soaked in the solution suggested by the manufacturer, or in equal parts of white vinegar and tap water for twenty minutes or so, then rinsed completely and dried. Meticulous care of pouches is an absolute necessity for the person with a urostomy. Emptying pouches frequently makes sense too, so that old urine never comes in contact with the opening of the stoma. Many pouches are made with some kind of anti-reflux mechanism so that urine is stored away from the stoma.

During the day when people stand or sit, gravity drains urine away from the stoma. During sleep, or other long bed rest, the bottom of the pouch is connected to tubing which attaches in turn to some kind of night drainage

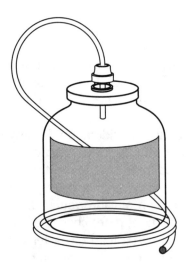

Night drainage system

system. This might be a large vinyl bag made for that purpose which hooks over the bed frame, or a large jug modified and placed on the floor inside a wastebasket, a beach bag or other covering. Gravity continues to keep urine away from the stoma so that infection can't get a toehold.

To avoid creating a vacuum in the system, which would prevent the easy flow of urine, a small amount of fluid is left in the pouch before connecting to the night drainage. Also, the tubing is secured at the top of the vented bottle so that no more than one inch (2.5 cm) or so of it extends into the bottle; should the level of urine rise above the bottom of the tubing, drainage stops.

People with a urostomy know that bacteria thrive in concentrated urine—so they drink *lots* of fluids (good advice for most people), at least eight or ten glasses a day. They never pass a drinking fountain without stopping! This keeps the urine dilute, and flowing swiftly away from the kidneys.

Too, they should learn the signs and symptoms of possible urinary tract infection and report for medical care *immediately* if any of these occur: fever, chills, flank or abdominal pain, bloody or tea-colored urine, foul smelling or "thick" whitish urine. (People with an ileal or a colonic conduit will normally have mucus in the urine, since the intestinal segment continues to secrete mucus; this should not be confused with pus and infection. There are products available to disperse thick mucus in the pouch.)

Regular check-ups include urinalysis and a blood test to see that the kidneys are functioning well. Doctors schedule periodic IVPs if the person tolerates them; otherwise different tests are used. It's a good idea to plan a long-term check-up schedule with the doctor.

The other fundamental concern for people with urostomies is the nature of urine and its flow. Urine flows everywhere. It wanders into the tiniest holes in the pouch seal.

Expert instruction on applying the pouch, appropriate skin preparation and protective products, and a properly-fitted appliance (followed by supervised practice, and then reasonable care in applying pouches) forestall most difficulties. Preventing irritation or healing it at the first hint of trouble is important.

If any of the skin around the stoma is not protected from urine, it can become thickened and tender. This overgrowth of skin is called *hyperplasia*; it often appears as a ring of "warty" skin around the stoma when the stoma opening of the pouch is too big. This means it's necessary to remeasure the stoma periodically (frequently at first when it is shrinking) and to cover *all* skin around the stoma.

Sometimes, urine which is alkaline forms scratchy, irritating crystals which encrust on and around the stoma. Making the urine more acid and using the proper opening diameter on the pouch prevents this *encrustation.* Two or three glasses of cranberry juice each day can make the urine more acid; surprisingly enough, orange juice or other citrus doesn't work, since it becomes alkaline in the body. Or the doctor may prescribe vitamin C tablets or another medication or may make other dietary suggestions.

People may want to test their urine at home periodically to find out its *pH*—how alkaline or acidic it is. With the pouch off, the person lets a little urine drip on the skin and dips a piece of *nitrazine* (litmus) paper into the fresh urine without touching the skin. Nitrazine paper, available through the pharmacy, changes color to show whether the urine is alkaline or acidic. For an accurate reading, the urine must be fresh and not from the pouch.

If encrustation does occur, the crystals can be dissolved with a solution of one part white vinegar to one part water. For ten minutes, three times a day, the person applies a washcloth or gauze pad soaked in the vinegar solution as a compress to the stoma or the skin where the crystals are. (Exposing the stoma for soaks is easier with some kinds of pouching systems than with others. In some cases, it may be advisable to switch temporarily to another type of appliance, such as a two-piece disposable system, where the pouch can be removed and reapplied simply.) In addition, a person can use a syringe (infant ear syringe, perhaps) to insert a half cup or so of vinegar solution through the valve into the empty pouch at bedtime. This lets the solution bathe the stoma—*if* it can reach the stoma; this does not work if the pouch is made with an anti-reflux construction to keep urine stored away from the stoma.

Urine contains dissolved minerals and some other substances which tend to form kidney stones in some people. Drinking abundant fluids, and, if the doctor recommends it, cutting down on certain foods, may solve this problem. (Which food to restrict depends on which minerals cause problems in a particular individual.)

The final concern of urine flow is that it's constant. At

first this may make keeping a dry area around the stoma while changing an appliance seem impossible, but there are such useful strategies as letting urine drip into the toilet, or using a tampon or wick of rolled gauze pressed against the stoma to catch urine drips while the skin is being washed, dried, and otherwise prepared for the pouch. (A pill bottle of proper size filled with gauze over the stoma is another possibility.) Some people swear that bending forward several times before removing the pouch "milks" the urine from the kidneys and ureters and helps the skin stay dry during the pouch change.

For the moment of pouch application, some people find it easier to keep a dry area around the stoma if they lie down or semi-recline in a chair, while others stand; a mirror is handy. Changing the pouch first thing in the morning before drinking anything, or at least a couple of hours after drinking, helps. It's important to change to a clean pouch at least once a week.

Since a urostomy is connected directly to organs essential for life, proper care is even more urgent than it is with other ostomies. But, that commitment made, a person can start *living* with a urostomy: working, playing, loving. No longer a urostomy which just happens to have a person attached, he or she can become a *person* who just happens to have a urostomy.

CHAPTER 12 ❧ *Pouches and the Skin They Touch*

[Skin is] one of the most interesting and mystic structures. . .that outer rampart which separates us from the rest of the universe, the sack which contains that juice or essence which is me, or which is you, a moat defensive against insects, poisons, germs. . . .
Dr. Logan Clendening

Not many years ago, a lady made her first visit to a stoma clinic—to ask where she could buy good rubber gloves, like "the kind they used to make." Thirty-five years before, when she had had her surgery, her nurse had suggested taping a rubber glove over the new stoma to collect the body waste. The woman had been doing it ever since, but she couldn't find any good rubber gloves anymore. She wept when she found out how many easier and better ways there are now.

Another ostomy patient startled his new doctor by displaying the collection device he'd developed and worn for some time: a cigar box, carefully waterproofed. There are several stories of people using a hot water bottle, slit to cover the stoma.

And only a few years ago, according to a story we were told, a delegate from India came to a UOA conference and was proud because he'd learned to cope with his ostomy—by taping an empty tuna fish can on his belly.

That a delegate could travel from India to the United States wearing a tuna fish can says something rather remarkable about human spirit and ingenuity. But it's infinitely easier to manage with a secure, comfortable, and inconspicuous pouch, a passport back to the normal world.

Pouch. Appliance. Bag. Whatever one calls it, it refers to the device, usually made of plastic or rubber, worn over the stoma to collect feces or urine as it is discharged, and to hold it until a convenient time for disposal. It's basically a thin-walled pouch that, when not in use, looks rather like an off-duty balloon.

What one calls it is a matter of personal preference. "Appliance" is a common term because the device is applied to the skin. Some people recoil from the term "bag"—while others sport T-shirts with "Bag Lady" or "I've got it in the bag" on them.

Whatever they are called, ostomy appliances aren't new. Probably the first ostomy pouch was a small leather bag designed in 1795 by a French surgeon, Daguesceau, for a patient on whom he had performed sigmoid colon surgery.

But until the late 1940s, with the coming of antibiotics, most surgeons shied away from ostomy surgery. The few patients who survived relied on bulky pads and dressings. One company supplied a cumbersome rubber appliance during the early 1900s.

The choice between smelly piles of dressings and heavy rubber appliances wasn't enough for the ever-increasing group of ostomy patients in the late 1940s and after. Now that surgeons were doing more surgeries, and many more people were surviving and expecting to resume a reasonably-normal life, demand was growing for lightweight, odor-resistant, secure coverings. Plastics entered the scene at about the same time.

Several old-line hospital supply companies began to develop special ostomy products and discovered they had stumbled onto a growth industry. Other ostomy pouches and supplies were developed and marketed by people who had ostomies themselves and who were frustrated in their own searches for something that really worked.

Now, the person who was once stymied by the lack of choices may be bewildered by the huge variety of appliances available: disposable, reusable, one-piece, two-piece, transparent, opaque, plain, fancy. The mind reels!

The goal is a pouch which fits properly, is comfortable, adheres well, is odor-proof, non-irritating to the skin, secure, economical and invisible under clothing and collects the output until a convenient time for emptying. It's a big order, but more and more people are finding the right appliance for themselves.

Some old-timers stick to an old favorite. Carol, for instance, really feels most comfortable with her sturdy black rubber, gas-valve appliance. Other people want to try everything. One ET nurse who has an ostomy is working his way through all the ileostomy pouches and combinations of equipment available, so that he can advise his clients better and increase his own comfort.

Basically, the kind of pouch depends on the kind of surgery, and the kind of person who has the ostomy. If the person has a urostomy, for instance, he or she needs an appliance to catch and hold a constant discharge of urine, and to protect the skin around the stoma from urine. A valve at the bottom keeps urine in the pouch and then releases it easily when the valve is opened for emptying. Special water-resistant adhesives hold the pouch securely in place.

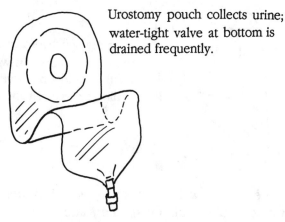

Urostomy pouch collects urine; water-tight valve at bottom is drained frequently.

The person with an ileostomy, with a liquid or semi-solid waste usually discharged at frequent times during the day, also needs a pouch which can be emptied easily. (Non-stick spray or a drop of mineral oil, placed in the bottom of a pouch after emptying and spread along the lower sides, makes it easier to empty later.) The drainage opening must be larger than the one on a urostomy pouch. Here the danger to the skin around the stoma comes from enzymes in the stool. Whatever holds the appliance to the skin need not be waterproof, but must protect the skin from enzyme damage.

The "drainable" pouch collects stool; bottom is closed securely with clamp or other closure device. Bottom opening must be large enough so feces can pass through it.

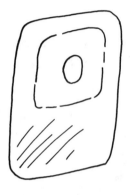

A security pouch for a colostomy collects any drainage between irrigation. It does not have a bottom opening but is small and compact.

The person with a colostomy who has loose and/or unpredictable stools needs the same kind of drainable pouch. This means patients with new colostomies and anyone with a colostomy made in the first two-thirds of the colon, or with loose stools for any reason (radiation therapy or chemotherapy, perhaps, or simply the 24-hour flu). Many people who choose not to irrigate also will want a drainable pouch that they can empty without having to remove it from the skin.

The person with ostomy surgery in the sigmoid colon eventually may have stool much like that before surgery. If he or she irrigates and has little or no discharge between irrigations, a soft square of absorbent material, perhaps with a plastic backing, can be used. For more security, others may choose a small closed pouch which is changed when the irrigation is done or a colostomy "plug" that fits into the stoma, blocking noise and odor. As long as the stool is fairly solid, it isn't likely to pool on the skin and injure it.

In fact, however, skin care is a major concern for anyone with an ostomy. As Katherine Jeter, ET, says: "The stoma will take care of itself; you must take care of your skin."

Why is it so important to keep the skin in top condition? Comfort, for one reason. Irritated, weepy skin *hurts*. Security is another motive. Healthy, smooth skin provides the ideal surface for a pouch, which may adhere poorly to rough, injured skin. Odor builds up also, when bacteria or other particles linger on irritated skin. Health is yet another factor; neither infected skin nor broken skin (which lets the wrong substances into and out of the body) is good for anyone.

Victor Alterescu, RN, ET, says "Your skin should be absolutely healthy underneath that pouch and should look just the same as it does anywhere else. Not like a football, not like a raw tomato, not like eggplant—nothing—just good healthy skin."

What can make the *peristomal skin*, the skin around the stoma, look like a raw tomato? Several things. This is plain old ordinary skin, but now it is being exposed to a rather extraordinary environment.

Enzymes from loose stool (from ileostomies and some colostomies) can digest skin as eagerly as they do food, leading to raw, "weeping" skin. Urine from a urostomy can damage the skin, leaving gray, "warty," thickened skin or encrustations of urine crystals.

The peristomal skin is injured when pouches are removed too often or too roughly. Very frequent pouch changes can strip off the surface layer skin cells faster than they can be replaced, causing redness and then more serious damage. As people get older, their skin gets drier and more fragile; this means that tape can stick more tenaciously and can pull off more skin cells when pouches are removed. For anyone, removing a pouch roughly can tear the skin. If body hair is ripped out as the pouch is taken off, the area becomes irritated. If the person wears a belt with a pouch, and cinches it too tightly, pressure sores can develop under the belt.

Allergic reactions to any ostomy product in contact with the peristomal skin can cause itching, redness, swelling and weeping of the skin. Perspiration, especially during hot weather or strenuous activity, can lead to heat rash on the skin under a plastic pouch.

All these conditions can cause raw areas, where the protective barrier of the skin is broken. Meanwhile, the warm, moist environment both in and underneath a pouch encourages bacteria and fungi (including yeast) to thrive. With a break in the epidermis, the outer layer of skin, these unwelcome invaders can get into the body and cause infection.

The good news is that, most of the time, these problems don't have to happen. *The person who wears an ostomy pouch can prevent most peristomal skin troubles by treating the skin gently and by keeping it clean and completely covered.* (All the "how-to" information is in *Chapter 13—Pouch Skills*.)

One of the major advances in protecting the skin around the stoma has been the *skin barrier*. Several years ago, Dr. Rupert Turnbull of the Cleveland Clinic accidentally spilled a container of *karaya* denture powder on himself. As he tried to clean his hands, he discovered that the karaya became a kind of mucilage when it was wet. Serendipity! Karaya, made from the sap of a species of tree from India, became the great-granddaddy of skin barriers for people with ostomies. Still used as powder, paste or solid sheet, it expands as heat from the body hits it and molds to the body surface, protecting the skin from enzymes or other harmful irritants and holding the pouch securely in place. Also, the person with a colostomy who removes pouches every day or so for irrigation can leave a skin barrier in place for several days, giving the surface layer of skin a chance to recover between pouch changes.

Manufacturers have developed many kinds of skin barriers, including thin pectin-based wafers or washers, transparent sheets of "breathable" plastic film, pastes and powders. An ET nurse is an excellent resource for finding out, for instance, which ones are water-soluble and won't work with a urostomy, or which ones are least likely to cause allergic reactions.

There are also wipes and sprays, called *skin sealants* or protectants. Sometimes these are used under skin barriers; they are especially helpful in protecting the surface layer of skin from frequent pouch changes. When these sealants are used, they need to dry thoroughly before anything is put over them.

Some people develop allergies to skin barriers, or to any of the products used with ostomies. For those with sensitive skin or allergies, a patch test is the safest way to experiment before using any new product near the stoma. (Directions are in *Chapter 13—Pouch Skills*.)

If the skin rebels, even after it's been treated with tender loving care, what then? For a mild problem, perhaps a little redness, one looks for the cause and removes it. Perhaps the pouch needs to be emptied more often— when it's about one-third full is just right—so it doesn't pull away from the skin and allow leakage. Or the peristomal area may be damaged from frequent pouch removals; a skin barrier left on the skin for several days will protect the skin until it heals.

First aid for minor problems involves cleaning the area well, drying it with extra care (perhaps with the "cool" or "low" setting on a portable hair dryer), and protecting all the peristomal skin with a skin barrier. Many of the wafer skin barriers will cling even to slightly-weepy skin and allow it to heal.

For anything more serious, the faster a person seeks the help of an ET nurse, the better.

✳✳✳✳✳

When Don Binder had his ileostomy surgery in 1959, there weren't any ET nurses around to advise him on the best kind of pouch. After a number of wild goose chases, "We went to a surgical supply dealer who showed us an appliance that didn't require cement. We bought it and I immediately put it on. Then we went to a supermarket, and as I was pushing the cart I felt the trickle on my leg. We later discovered that what we had bought was a colostomy irrigating dome which had no protection for the skin. The salesperson didn't know the difference nor did I. Fortunately, that doesn't happen very often these days."

Getting the right pouching system, essential as it is, presents challenges. If the stoma protrudes enough and is regularly-shaped on a reasonably-flat surface, away from prominent bones or scars, on a fairly slender abdomen, almost any pouch should adhere well. But anatomy isn't the only factor in choosing a pouch. It's also important to think about finances, sharpness of vision, dexterity, overall energy and mobility, amount of ostomy output, lifestyle, and personal preferences. The athlete, the young child who outgrows pouches faster than shoes, the older person with very dry skin—in fact everyone, for some reason or other, has special needs when it comes to equipment choices. Considering how important the right pouch is, it would be a blessing if everyone had access to advice from an ET nurse or from another health professional who is knowledgeable about ostomies.

There are many ways to get a bird's-eye view of what equipment is available. Most UOA chapters have a display board of different kinds of pouches and other ostomy supplies. Ads in the *Ostomy Quarterly*, a visit to a pharmacy or surgical supply house which stocks pouches, or word-of-mouth can all be helpful. These are also good sources for finding out about such related equipment as pouch covers (whether breathable white cotton for comfort and the prevention of heat rash, or fancy); hole cutters to make stoma openings in skin barrier wafers; or assorted gadgets for centering the pouch over the stoma.

Pouches can be disposable (made to be discarded after one use, usually a few days), or reusable (washed and then used again, many times). Using disposables regularly may cost more money but saves cleaning time. The used pouch, wrapped securely in aluminum foil, an opaque plastic bag, or other odor-proof covering is thrown in the trash; most are not made to be flushed down the toilet.

The person who relies on reusable pouches usually has two or three. While one is being worn, another is being soaked, dried, and aired. Special cleaning/soaking solutions, which clean, deodorize, and maintain ostomy appliances, can be purchased from the appliance supplier. (There are specific products to clean urostomy pouches and dissolve crystals left by urine.) After the pouch has been soaked, the inside can be scrubbed with an appliance cleaning brush or a baby-bottle brush.

Disposable pouches come in one-piece or two-piece styles. The one-piece pouches come with tape and/or a piece of skin barrier bonded to the pouch. These all-in-one pouches can be very quick and easy to apply, a plus for many people, including those with arthritis in their hands or other limitations in dexterity. Many one-piece pouches have belt tabs, and some incorporate a gas-release valve. (A separate skin barrier wafer, cut to fit around the stoma, can be used, if needed, under the pouch. This is a useful technique for the person with an irregularly-shaped stoma who wants to use a pouch with a precut round stoma opening. Also, the pouch can be disposed of and a new pouch applied, without removing the barrier, which can be helpful in preventing skin damage from frequent appliance changes.) There are some one-piece styles available with a cut-to-fit stoma opening.

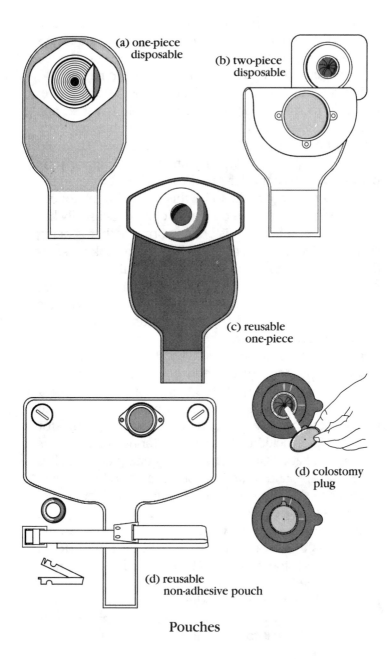

(a) one-piece
disposable

(b) two-piece
disposable

(c) reusable
one-piece

(d) colostomy
plug

(d) reusable
non-adhesive pouch

Pouches

Two-piece disposable appliances come with a skin barrier piece that adheres to the skin and a second pouch piece that can be attached and removed readily. Some of these have a pouch with a flange which snaps onto a corresponding rim on a pliable skin barrier wafer (rather like a "Tupperware^R" seal). These two-piece systems mean that the pouch can be removed (for showering, perhaps, for colostomy irrigation, or just for a thorough pouch cleaning) without disturbing the skin barrier. Some can be "burped" to release gas: The person opens the seal above the stoma a little bit and closes it again after the gas is gone. Some two-piece systems have a skin barrier with a "floating" or "accordion" flange, especially comfortable for the person with a new stoma and a tender abdomen. With this, the thumb is placed *under* the flange and supports it while the pouch is being snapped on so that there is no pressure on the abdomen.

The person with a colostomy might choose a "colostomy plug" two-piece system. This includes a faceplate which adheres to the skin and a snap-on cap with an attached soft plastic foam plug. The flexible plug, inserted a short way into the stoma, blocks stool and minimizes noise; gas is dispersed continuously through a deodorizing filter. While some people (usually those who irrigate) use this system all the time, it can also be a useful alternative for short periods for those who don't irrigate, with a regular pouch snapped onto the faceplate the rest of the time.

Reusable appliances come in adhesive (made to be stuck to the skin) and non-adhesive styles. The adhesive pouch may have a faceplate already bonded to the pouch. If the pouch is separate, it is attached to the faceplate with a locking device supplied by the manufacturer, a double-faced adhesive seal, or cement. The faceplate can be adhered either directly to the skin, often with a special cement, or to a wafer or washer of skin barrier which then sticks to the skin. Manufacturers can custom-make the faceplate to fit the person with special needs; other people may prefer the sturdier materials of reusable pouches or find them less costly to use.

Some people favor a non-adhesive reusable pouch. These are made with a silicone "doughnut" around the stoma opening of the pouch. The skin around the stoma gradually conforms to the "doughnut," making a channel around the stoma. A belt holds the pouch in place. The pouches are easily removed and replaced and ordinarily are used without skin barriers or adhesives.

What about the person who doesn't have the ideal stoma perfectly situated on a flat abdomen? With help from an ET nurse or other knowledgeable person, he or she learns to build up a flat area around the stoma, using skin barrier paste or small pieces of skin barrier wafer cut to fit the dips and crannies under the pouch. This is especially important if these irregularities occur right next to the stoma where urine or stool can pool and leak. A skin barrier wafer can be cut to compensate for an irregularly-shaped stoma or a stoma placed too close to a bone or scar. (Custom-made reusable faceplates are another option.)

Some short, flush, or retracted stomas don't cause problems with standard pouches. Sometimes, however, urine or feces tends to pool around the stoma, undermine pouches, and injure the skin. What is needed is a way to get a very tight seal on the skin right next to the stoma and, if possible, to help the stoma protrude a bit above skin level so that it can act as a spigot, directing the stool or urine into the pouch. *Convexity* in a pouch system does this, curving firmly against the skin right around the stoma, creating a tighter seal and pushing the stoma out somewhat.

This convex curve is built into the faceplates of some ready-made pouches, both disposable and reusable; some companies also custom-fit a convex reusable faceplate.

Convexity

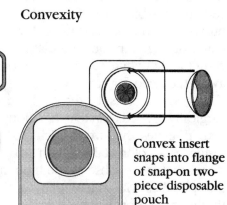

Convex insert snaps into flange of snap-on two-piece disposable pouch

Pouch with convexity built into faceplate

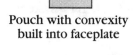

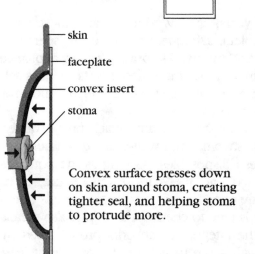

skin

faceplate

convex insert

stoma

Convex surface presses down on skin around stoma, creating tighter seal, and helping stoma to protrude more.

Convex inserts, stiff curved pieces of plastic that snap into certain skin barrier wafers, are another possibility. ET nurses can demonstrate different techniques for achieving convexity. (A very flexible plastic film skin barrier may cling tightly enough to the skin around a flush stoma to avoid the need for convexity.)

Sometimes it is better to have a "difficult" stoma surgically revised than to suffer along for months or years with pouches that won't stick and skin problems. For instance, a colorectal surgeon may be able to move a stoma that is too close to the hipbone to another site so that pouches will adhere well. Or the person with continuing pouch problems because of a hernia around the stoma or a retracted stoma may want to consult a surgeon rather than "making do" with makeshift pouching systems.

*****

Until recent years, ostomy odor was an almost insurmountable problem, a frequent source of whispers and non-acceptance. Now, thanks to advances in appliance materials and more trustworthy deodorants, odor is seldom a problem, although it may take a little trial and error to find what works best.

Cleanliness is the basis of any attack on unwanted odors: baths or showers and well-cleaned reusable appliances, or fresh disposables. As long as the pouch is intact and closed and the skin seal is secure, there shouldn't be any odor. This means that if there is unexpected odor, it is time to check for a leak. It also means not breaking the integrity of an odor-proof pouch by puncturing it with a pin to get the gas out (or at least resealing any puncture with non-porous tape).

Many pouches are made either to disperse gas continuously through a built-in deodorizing patch, or to hold it until there's privacy to release it through the bottom, out a special valve, or through a "burping" technique; this gets rid of "bag bulge." Using a wick or spray deodorant or lighting a match in the room (as long as there's no oxygen nearby) takes care of the gas odor. Although many appliances are now so odor-proof that no deodorant is necessary, a number of ostomy suppliers offer effective deodorants. For instance, a few drops or a tablet in the pouch (when it's opened, rinsed, or changed) suffice. Some people depend on oral deodorants taken as a tablet, liquid, or powder on a regular daily basis. (While these are effective, some may have possible side effects and their use should be discussed with the doctor or ET nurse.) The ET nurse also has expert advice on the best ways to deal with odor if special problems arise.

From experience, people discover that some foods increase odor in feces or urine. This is a highly individual matter, so a little detective work is necessary. Parsley and yogurt, used liberally in the diet, are recommended by many as good natural ways to control odor. (See *Chapter 15—Eating Well.*)

Many people with ostomies tend to be hypersensitive about the possibility of odor and fret too much about "offending." (In fact, stool and passed gas from anyone, with or without an ostomy, smells about the same.) However, some people, often older people, may lose some or all of their sense of smell. They need to be particularly careful with pouch and skin cleanliness and may want to check in periodically with an ET nurse (or with a helpful relative or friend with intact sense of smell) to be sure that their appliance is odor-free.

Noise, both of the pouch and of passing gas, is another concern. Manufacturers now make appliances from quiet, non-rustling materials to make pouch noise minimal. The person who begins to pass gas can stop the noise by placing the forearm firmly against the stoma. (It takes a little practice to learn to do this effectively but casually.)

Ignoring any noise, laughing about it—or just accepting it—are other options.

Ostomy equipment can be expensive. Medicare, Medicaid, and some insurance programs cover some or all of the cost of ostomy supplies in the U.S. To ensure proper credit, ostomy products should be described as "prosthetic appliances." When money is a problem, there are ways to reduce costs without skimping on care: checking whether each product used is really necessary— in fact, simplifying pouching systems isn't a bad idea for anyone—or cutting skin barrier wafers diagonally into two pieces so that they last through twice as many pouch changes, and so on. Those who irrigate might use squares cut from disposable diapers rather than pouches, and *everyone* can save money by comparison shopping. (Some people have become exceedingly ingenious at saving dollars!) An ET nurse or UOA meeting can offer other suggestions.

It's worthwhile for anyone with an ostomy to find a pharmacy or appliance source which is really interested in and well-informed about ostomy supplies. Some of the large mail order firms which have been in business a long time are able and willing to offer personalized advice. For those with a special problem, some companies specialize in custom appliances.

The good old days? They weren't all that good for people with ostomies—and the appliance companies, which have produced booklets, slide shows and films on ostomy care, along with a continuing stream of new pouches and skin care products, can take much of the credit for the enormous strides forward in a very few years.

Virginia Pearce looks back a few decades at the days after her ileostomy: "Several *weeks* after surgery the long awaited appliance arrived. . .a COLOSTOMY pouch with a wire frame that protruded out about an inch. When I was first told about this 'ileostomy' and having to wear a 'bag', I decided that my life would be spent in maternity smocks, and when THAT appliance was presented to me, I *knew* I was going to look pregnant for the next 30 or 40 years.

"But the worst was yet to come. This pouch had no bottom opening, a three-inch stoma opening and was held on by belts and buckles, no cement or skin barrier. When I sat up in the wheelchair my tummy was concave (hard to believe now) and warm, brown fluid trickled down my abdomen. . .ah! the good old days!

"Determined there must be a *better* appliance somewhere, I got a pass from the hospital, hired a cab, and went to the biggest surgical supply house in Salt Lake City.

"The sales person showed me the only alternative appliance he had. There was a metal ring (with a two inch opening) and over the ring you put latex rubber pouches which went inside a white satin cover. The purpose of the lovely satin cover was to keep the thin rubber pouch from elongating as it filled up. The appliance had a wide belt and buckles—no cement. Very often when you sat down, with a partially filled pouch, everything 'pooched up' and over, and there was that nice brown stain again!. . . .

"Ah, the good old days!"

CHAPTER 13 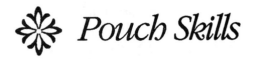 *Pouch Skills*

Practice is nine-tenths.
Ralph Waldo Emerson

Living with an ostomy often involves learning how to take care of an external pouch and the skin it touches. These new skills take some practice, but are not difficult. Doing them correctly saves time, supplies, and the peristomal skin—and makes one's life much easier!

CLOSING DRAINABLE POUCHES

Drainable pouches come with some kind of clamp or other closure device. If directions come with the device, they are the best source of information about how to open and close it.

A common basic clamp has a single bar attached at one end to an envelope-like second arm. To close the pouch, hold the open clamp at the hinge, and place the single bar of the clamp about an inch from the outlet of the drainable pouch. The bottom of the pouch is folded over the single bar *once only*, and the envelope arm is pressed firmly over the single bar until it locks in place. (If the bottom of the pouch is folded over more than once, the

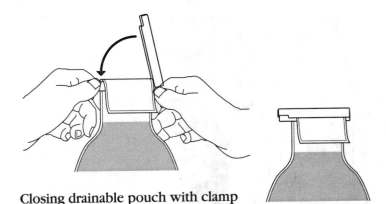

Closing drainable pouch with clamp

clamp often doesn't lock properly.)

If necessary, drainable pouches can be closed with a rubber band.

EMPTYING THE POUCH

When the pouch is about one-third full, it's time to empty it into the toilet. You will need tissue or wipes to clean the pouch outlet after emptying. Some people also like to have a cup or large syringe of water handy to rise the inside of the pouch after emptying.

You can sit on or can face the toilet so that the pouch is over the toilet bowl. Before emptying the pouch, hold up the bottom of the pouch so that the stool or urine moves away from the outlet, remove the closure device or open the valve, and put the closure device (if any) somewhere close by, where it can be retrieved easily.

Some people like to fold the end of a drainable pouch back on itself, making a short cuff (about an inch or 2.5 cm) before emptying. The cuffed area then stays clean.

To prevent splashing of stool, you can float a "raft" of folded tissue in the bowl before opening the clamp, or

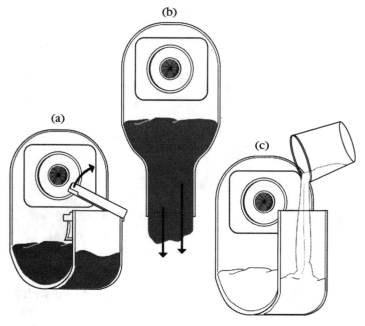

(b)

(a)

(c)

Emptying the pouch

can flush the toilet while aiming the outlet of the pouch
into the toilet and emptying it.

To drain feces, use thumb and fingers outside the
pouch, squeezing contents out into the toilet bowl.

It's optional to hold the pouch outlet up again, add a
few ounces of water, swish it around the pouch, and then
empty the pouch contents again into the toilet.

Wipe the bottom of the pouch and/or uncuff it, adding
a drop or tablet of commercial pouch deodorant at this
point to a drainable pouch, if desired. (There should be
no aspirin tablets or alcohol-based mouthwashes in the
pouch; they may help odor but can injure the stoma.) The
pouch is then closed with the valve or clamp.

Valve-bottom (urostomy) pouches don't get rinsed or
deodorized, but the valve area needs to be cleaned very
carefully to prevent odor.

CHANGING A POUCH

It's important to change the ostomy pouch down to the skin on a regular schedule so that the skin and stoma can be cleaned thoroughly and checked for any problems. This cuts down on leaks and makes emergency pouch changes less likely.

But how often? That depends on the person and the ostomy. Most people whose ostomies are not managed with irrigation should be able to go at least three days between changes. Many people put on a fresh pouch every five to seven days. The "extended wear" skin barriers let some people go two weeks or even longer between changes.

If there is a leak, the pouch must be changed immediately; patching does not work. Sometimes, a leak is only under the skin barrier, where the peristomal skin will start to itch, burn, or hurt. This still needs to be changed right away to avoid skin damage.

The best time to change a pouch is when the ostomy is least active. Often this is early in the morning in conjunction with a shower.

1. Assembling Supplies. When it's time to change a pouch, all the necessary supplies are assembled first: to remove the used pouch, and to dispose of it or clean it later; to measure the stoma, if necessary; to clean the peristomal area; and to put together the particular pouching system and adhere it to the skin. This process seems complicated at first, but it gets easier with practice. Keeping all needed supplies together in a box or in an area of the cupboard may be helpful.

Some people with more complicated appliance systems do any pouch assembly well before time for a change. Then they simply remove the used pouch, take a bath or shower, and put on the already-prepared fresh pouch.

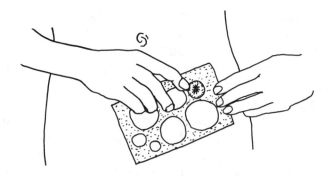

2. Measuring the Stoma. Once the stoma has reached a fairly stable size (after a few months), it needs to be measured only a few times a year, unless there's a marked weight change. During the first weeks after surgery, the stoma keeps changing; measuring is done with every pouch change at first, and then less and less frequently.

Pouch manufacturers supply measuring guides with cut-out circles of different diameters for measuring the stoma for the correct-size pouch. The smallest cut-out ring which fits comfortably around the base of the stoma without touching it is used to order the pouch size, following the manufacturer's directions.

The right size opening for the pouch is crucial. Any rigid edges need to be a bit larger than the stoma, with about a 1/16 to 1/8 inch (1.5-3 mm) clearance all around. This protects most of the peristomal skin, but still gives the stoma a little room to expand when it is discharging waste. without being pinched or cut. This is critical because, since the stoma doesn't have any sensory nerves, it can't signal if it's being injured.

The measuring guide can also be used as a pattern for cut-to-fit stoma openings on pouches or skin barrier wafers. As always, any rigid edge (like the plastic edge of a pouch) must be cut a little larger than the stoma. Skin barrier wafers with "give" to them can be cut to fit the stoma exactly, so that they cover all the skin around the stoma.

If a wafer skin barrier is correctly fitted under a pouch so that *all* the peristomal skin is protected, the pouch stoma opening can be almost any size as long as it's not too small.

Those who have irregularly-shaped stomas can make their own patterns from a sturdy card labeled "top" and "bottom," "right" and "left." This template is practice-fitted around the stoma until it is the correct shape, and then can be used as long as the stoma size and shape remain the same. (The card can be reinforced with tape to make it last longer.)

3. Removing the Used Pouch. This is done *gently* to protect the skin around the stoma. First the pouch is emptied and the clamp, if any, is put where it won't get lost. Rather than removing the pouch from the skin, one eases the skin from the pouch, working fingers and/or a wet swab between pouch and skin to break the seal, and supporting the skin until the pouch is off.

If cement has been used to adhere the pouch to the skin, an adhesive remover is applied to the area at the edge of the pouch. When the cement has been dissolved in that area, the loosened section of the pouch is freed from the skin. This process is repeated until the pouch is off.

The soiled pouch is set aside for cleaning, or put into an opaque plastic bag or aluminum foil for disposal; wrapping it in newspaper and placing it in a clear plastic bag is another option. These make odor-proof, see-through-proof coverings for disposal.

Removing used pouch

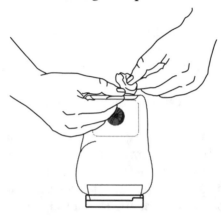

4. Cleaning Area Around Stoma. If possible, one chooses a time when the ostomy is "quiet" to change the pouch (before breakfast is a good time for many people). A shower, bath, or sponge bath with warm water usually cleans the area well, and water does not get into the stoma. Commercial products designed specifically for cleaning the peristomal skin are available; these are effective, but not essential for most people. If mild soap is used (without oils, perfumes, or other additives), it must be rinsed off gently but completely. Using a small amount of baking soda in the water is an option if the skin is a little irritated or itchy.

The skin is then patted dry. Some traces of adhesive or skin barrier can be safely left on the skin; that's better than rubbing too briskly to remove them. A dry cloth or gauze is much better than water for taking off some skin barriers.

If the stoma continues discharging during the cleaning process, a washcloth, gauze pad or toilet tissue can catch any waste; for urine, a tampon or gauze wick pressed over the stoma opening, or a pill bottle with cotton balls in it can help keep the skin dry during cleaning.

Cleaning area around stoma

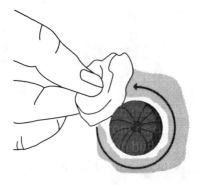

5. Applying Skin Barrier. Many people rely on some kind of commercial skin barrier to protect the skin around the stoma, and many disposable pouches have some kind of skin barrier already attached. If a wafer needs to be cut to fit, the pattern is followed with small scissors with curved blades. Cookie cutter-like devices to punch out the correct-sized opening are also available. However it is done, any cut edge that will hug the stoma needs to be smooth, with no jagged edges that could injure the stoma. A squeeze of skin barrier paste can protect any uncovered skin right around the stoma; a moistened finger applies it.

Some skin barriers should be moistened before applying. Some wafers stick better if they are warmed between the hands for a minute or so before the paper backing is removed. Directions for application of the various skin barrier products appear on each container or in a package insert.

Skin barriers (or pouches) adhere best to a smooth, level surface. Body hair on the peristomal skin can be clipped with small scissors or shaved with an electric razor. (A safety razor tends to nick the skin, which can cause problems under a pouch.) To level the surface (especially

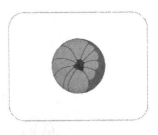

Applying skin barrier

important right next to the stoma), skin barrier paste or a small extra piece of skin barrier wafer can fill in any little dips.

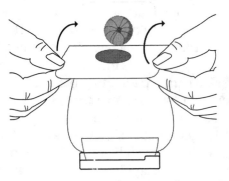

Putting on clean pouch

6. Putting on a Clean Pouch. If there is an opening at the bottom of the pouch, it is closed. The front and back pieces of the pouch are separated to avoid creating a vacuum (blowing in a small puff of air is one way to do this). If a pouching system has several components, they can be ssembled first; the entire system is then applied.

Any backing paper is peeled away, carefully and smoothly, either before or while the pouch is being pressed to the abdomen with no air pockets. Most people start at the bottom of the pouch before applying the sides and top, so that they can see that the pouch opening is centered over the stoma.

One can stand, sit or semi-recline in a chair, or lie down while doing this, as long as the abdominal surface around the stoma is kept as flat as possible. A mirror (possibly a magnifying mirror) can be helpful.

If there are problems centering the pouch opening over the stoma, there are ways to make it easier. For instance, applying only the skin barrier piece from a two-piece system makes it easy to see that the opening is correctly centered before the pouch is snapped on. Or a paper guide strip, rolled like the link in a paper chain, is placed into the stoma opening of the skin barrier flange or the pouch and then aligned over the stoma; the strip passes through the flange or falls into the pouch as the piece is pressed into place.

After the pouch is attached, it's worth spending several seconds pressing it to the skin, paying special attention to the area right around the stoma.

If cement is used, a *thin* coat is applied to both the faceplate and to a circle of skin around the stoma, slightly larger than the area the faceplate will cover. (Tape will cover the area beyond the faceplate.) The cement dries for a few minutes before the faceplate (usually with the pouch already attached) is secured to the skin. It's crucial to allow enough drying time for the solvents (which keep the cement spreadable) to evaporate, so they will not be trapped under the faceplate and cause skin irritation.

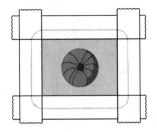

Applying tape

7. Using Tape and/or Belt. Many disposable pouches now come with an attached rim of tape. For those that don't, many people like the extra security of picture-framing the pouch with four strips of tape, usually a porous tape that lets the skin breathe. (Waterproof tape can be added for bathing or swimming.)

Some people add a belt. The belt is worn around the hips at the level of the stoma, and is loose enough so that two fingers can be slipped easily between belt and skin. Many pouches or faceplates have tabs for a belt, or there are belts available (narrow to several inches wide) which can be worn without belt tabs.

8. Cleaning Up. The used disposable pouch can be wrapped and thrown away. (Most pouches are not made to be flushed down the toilet.) The reusable pouch can be cleaned with a commercially-available cleaning/soaking solution, or with liquid detergent with a small amount of bleach added. Cool water is preferable, since hot water tends to seal in odors. For urostomy pouches, a vinegar-water solution or ostomy appliance decrystalizer works to remove odor, bacteria, and crystals. The clean pouch can be air-dried. A bent wire clothes hanger will keep the

the pouch front and back separated for complete airing.

Cleaning up afterwards makes for a more pleasant environment—and is common courtesy if others use the area.

PATCH TESTING

The person with sensitive skin or allergies can patch test small samples of ostomy products (skin barrier, for instance) before using them near the stoma. If a peristomal skin irritation arises, a patch test may help determine whether allergy to a product is to blame.

For a patch test, a small quantity of the substance in question is applied to skin away from the stoma, taped in place, and left for 48 hours.

If there is any burning, itching, or other discomfort during the 48 hours, the sample is taken off immediately. Otherwise, the substance is removed after 48 hours; the site is checked for redness or rash half an hour later (after the normal irritation from the tape removal has subsided), and again 48 hours later, in case there's a delayed reaction. Sometimes the reaction is to the tape; when that happens, the redness occurs right where the tape was.

If there's no irritation, the product should be safe to use near the stoma. Allergy may develop after long use of a product, but what appears to be an allergic reaction is often irritation from the product rubbing against the skin.

CHAPTER 14 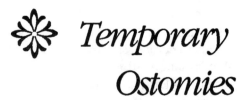 *Temporary Ostomies*

Life must be lived as we go along.
Robert J. Hastings

The best thing about temporary ostomies—aside from the fact that they save lives—is that they buy time while keeping future options open. They buy time during which a person can get healthier, or just bigger. They buy time for a surgical site beyond the ostomy to mend. Sometimes they buy time so that a person can be comfortable even if a cure isn't possible.

There are some things about temporary ostomies that aren't so good. Frequently there's no opportunity for psychological or physical preparation. The stoma(s) often must be created in haste and can be difficult to manage.

But perhaps the worst thing is that it is so very easy (and so natural) for the person with a temporary ostomy to put his or her life "on hold." Two months, six months, a year, or much longer can pass while the person waits. . .waits for the surgery to reconnect the digestive or urinary tract.

A "temporary" ostomy is one intended for a limited

period of time, of course—but it has another, more technical definition. In ostomy parlance, a colostomy or ileostomy is considered temporary if the lower part of the rectum and all of the anus are not removed. Potentially, then, the digestive tract still can be reconnected so that stool passes through the anus again (even though all or part of the colon may be missing). A urostomy is temporary if the bladder remains.

Who get temporary ostomies? Why?

Liz arrives in the emergency room with a ruptured bowel after a car accident. When she regains consciousness, she finds a large pouch on her belly. Her colostomy means that stool can exit the body before it reaches the damaged area; meanwhile, the injuries have a chance to heal.

Steve was always the healthiest and fittest of young men—until he developed the raging bloody diarrhea of acute ulcerative colitis. After almost two months in a hospital room, during which doctors tried every known nonsurgical treatment to tame his bowel, Steve got the word: The colon has to come out.

Although Steve was too sick for the lengthy operation necessary to construct some kind of internal reservoir (a possibility for a patient with ulcerative colitis), his surgeon was able to leave the fairly-healthy rectum and the anus in place to keep Steve's options open. With his diseased colon gone and a temporary ileostomy so that stool can exit his body, Steve has time to get healthy again and to consider his next step.

His temporary urostomy doesn't faze young Peter, celebrating a first birthday his parents feared he would never see. Born with a serious defect in his urinary tract, he needs to grow bigger before the defect can be surgically corrected. It will be a wait of several years, but Petey doesn't care how his urine exits his body. Now, if he can just reach some of that cake frosting. . .

Temporary Ostomies 145

Mrs. Wood is also celebrating a birthday, her 75th. Colorectal cancer, detected late, has blocked her bowel. Because the cancer has spread and her general health is poor, she isn't a candidate for the long surgery necessary to construct a permanent colostomy. But her surgeon can make her much more comfortable by constructing a "temporary" ostomy so that stool can exit her body before it reaches the obstruction.

What happens now for these people with temporary ostomies?

Liz loathes her ostomy: "Maybe it did save my life, but I wish I had died in the wreck rather than having to live with the thing." She curses the bulky stoma, awkwardly placed. It seems as if every time she bends, the bag loosens and leaks. Clothing? Designer jeans have given way to smocks (dark printed ones that don't show the stains). Friends? "Forget it. I wouldn't let *anyone* see me like this."

With Liz's slapdash care, the skin around the stoma has become red and weepy. She doesn't see any point in checking with an ET nurse (the ostomy professional) for help: "Why? It's just for a little longer." She's counting off the weeks (days? hours?) until her reconnection surgery when she can get rid of "it." *Then* she'll start living again. . .

Steve, on the other hand, is doing "great, thank you!" He's recovering from his major bout of ulcerative colitis and surgery, and faces more surgery in the next few months. But, minus a sick colon, he's beginning to feel healthier, even (sometimes) downright energetic. He can *eat*, he's gaining weight, and each day he increases the time he spends on the exercise bike and the distance he walks. He's *home* and, for the first time in months, he can believe in a future for himself. Steve doesn't love his ostomy—he finds it a real nuisance at times—but he tolerates it and takes good care of the skin around the stoma. (In fact, he's rather proud of himself for learning how to apply a pouch so well.) Because his surgeon projects at least a six-month wait before the next surgery, Steve plans a short vacation and then a return to part-time work in the interim. Before surgery, he couldn't get out of bed by himself. Now the challenge is to keep from overdoing. . . .

Little Petey doesn't care a bit about his temporary urostomy. He's healthy, content, and into everything. His parents realize that "temporary" is a relative term when applied to Pete's ostomy: "Temporary" means "for years." Sometimes they feel grateful. Other times, they can't stop looking ahead to the time when Pete's ostomy will be just a memory. Then. . .

Mrs. Wood is delighted (most of the time, anyway) with the "temporary" ostomy that she will have for the rest of her life. It has brought her freedom from the pain that was stalking her. *Now* she can do the things she loves to do: walk, visit with friends, read, crochet. . .

Everyone reacts differently to a temporary ostomy. One factor is what the "before" was like. For instance, the person with months of severe inflammatory bowel disease or excruciating cancer pain may welcome a temporary ostomy because "after" is so much better than "before." Another factor is how easily one can care for the ostomy (particularly the stoma and the skin around it). That depends not only on how the stoma is constructed but also on how well the person is instructed in stoma care. There are other factors, of course, because individuals *are* individuals and not cookie-cutter people.

Surgeons construct more temporary ostomies than permanent ones. In a temporary ostomy, as with a permanent one, part of the digestive or urinary tract is connected to the skin so that stool or urine will have an exit from the body.

For years, temporary ostomies have been used to bypass trauma, blockage, or birth defect in the colon or urinary tract. Another reason for making a temporary ostomy is to protect a fresh surgical site beyond the ostomy. (For instance, a temporary ostomy is frequently part of the alternative surgical procedures for ulcerative colitis, such as the ileoanal anastomosis with reservoir.) Surgeons have different ways of constructing the temporary ileostomy or colostomy, depending on the reason for the ostomy and on how much (if any) of the digestive tract needs to be removed. However the ostomy is made, there must be a stoma at the end of the functioning (food-digesting) intestinal tract to discharge stool. In addition, there has to be some provision for the bypassed intestine beyond the stoma. Like the village that becomes a ghost town after the traffic flow is diverted, this section of intestine is still there, but separated from the activity.

If part of the intestine is being bypassed for a time, but nothing needs to be removed, the surgeon can construct a *loop ostomy*, either an ileostomy or a colostomy. The intestine isn't cut in two, but a small part of it is pulled through an incision in the abdomen. A plastic rod (or perhaps a "bridge" made of body tissue) placed under the exposed piece of bowel keeps the "loop" of intestine from slipping back into the abdomen during the first several days after surgery. When healing has progressed enough so that the stoma won't slip back, any plastic device is removed.

Meanwhile, the loop of bowel is cut partway open (but not severed) during surgery and, it forms one large stoma with two openings. One opening is still connected to the functioning digestive tract and so it continues to pass stool. The second opening, the *mucous fistula*, is the beginning of the bypassed tube of intestine that ends at the anus. This bypassed intestine still produces mucus to lubricate itself; some of this may come through the mucous fistula and some through the anus. No more stool passes through the mucous fistula, unless there's some that didn't get cleaned out before surgery, or perhaps a bit that "migrates"

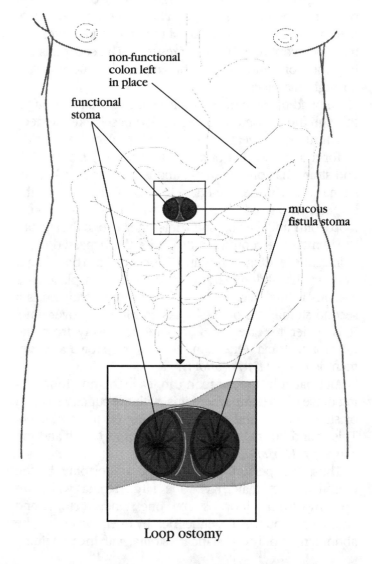

non-functional
colon left
in place

functional
stoma

mucous
fistula stoma

Loop ostomy

Temporary Ostomies *149*

over the stoma from one opening to the other. This large stoma is stitched or stapled to the skin.

Often the surgeon needs to cut the intestine in two, perhaps because a segment must be removed. After severing the bowel and, if necessary, taking out a diseased or injured segment, the surgeon has two entirely separate pieces left. The first, still part of the functioning intestinal tract, will continue to discharge stool. The second is the bypassed piece leading to the anus; only mucus passes through this piece.

The end of the functioning intestine is usually brought through the abdomen, folded back on itself like the neck of a turtleneck sweater and stitched in place on the skin to form an "end" (as opposed to a "loop") stoma. This end stoma has one opening, and is the standard kind of stoma found in permanent ostomies. (On occasion, the surgeon who needs to cut the bowel in two may make a loop stoma and then sever the intestine beyond the stoma.)

Then the surgeon must deal with the bypassed piece of intestine leading to the anus. The cut end can be brought through the abdominal wall and stitched in place as a mucous fistula. What it looks like on the abdomen is a second stoma; this often shrinks considerably over time. It is easier to care for if it is located away from the functional stoma. One name for this two-stoma arrangement is *double-barrel ostomy*.

Alternatively, the surgeon can leave the non-functioning piece of intestine where it is, with the cut end stitched or stapled shut, and with no opening on the abdomen. This "blind alley" is called a *Hartmann's pouch* and the surgery a *Hartmann's procedure*.

Thus, the person with a temporary ostomy in the digestive tract may have one large stoma with two openings from a loop ostomy; one standard stoma and another mucous fistula, either nearby or elsewhere on the abdomen; or only one standard stoma, with the remaining

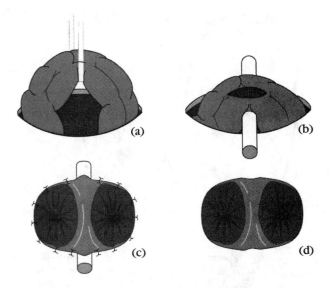

CONSTRUCTING A LOOP OSTOMY. The bowel is (a) brought through the abdominal wall, (b) supported temporarily by a rod or other device, and (c) opened. (d) After several days the rod is removed. One opening discharges stool, the other, mucus.

digestive tract a "blind alley" Hartmann's pouch within the abdomen. There are several reasons for the surgeon's choice of what kind of temporary ostomy to make, including how much surgery the patient can tolerate, whether part of the bowel needs to be removed, and how important it is that there be no possibility of stool migrating into the bypassed segment of intestine.

The other kind of temporary ostomy by which stool leaves the digestive tract is a *cecostomy*. A plastic or rubber tube is placed through a slit in the lower abdomen into the cecum, the cul-de-sac of bowel which forms the first part of the large intestine. The cecostomy tube then drains feces, quite liquid at this stage in its journey through the digestive tract, into a drainage bag. A cecostomy is used

DOUBLE-BARREL OSTOMY — two stomas

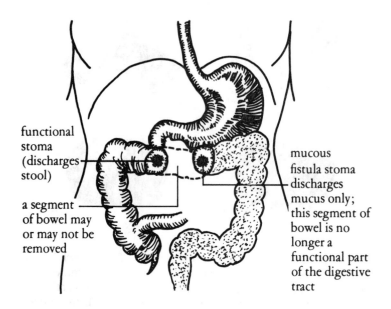

functional stoma (discharges stool)

mucous fistula stoma discharges mucus only; this segment of bowel is no longer a functional part of the digestive tract

a segment of bowel may or may not be removed

occasionally in an attempt to relieve blockage farther on in the colon or for a few days after major bowel surgery to remove gas before the intestines start working again. (Colorectal surgeons use the technique only rarely because they find that it often doesn't give satisfactory results.)

Temporary urinary tract diversions for both adults and children also include those in which a tube is inserted through the skin directly into the bladder and then drains urine into a drainage bag. Or, if there's an obstruction in the urine flow as it leaves the kidney and enters the ureter, a nephrostomy tube placed in the kidney allows urine to exit the body.

With children especially, temporary urinary diversions may bring one or both ureters through the skin in loop ureterostomies; nothing is severed and, as in digestive tract loop ostomies, the stoma has one functional and one

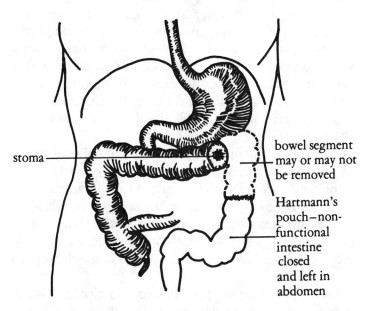

stoma

bowel segment
may or may not
be removed

Hartmann's
pouch—non-
functional
intestine
closed
and left in
abdomen

non-functional opening. There are several kinds of urinary diversions which leave all or part of the bladder intact. Potentially, in time, the urinary tract can be reconnected so that urine flows out of the body through the urethra; this surgery is called *undiversion.*

Physical care for the temporary ostomy, and especially for the surrounding skin can be either simple or quite challenging. A "good" stoma is fairly round and regular, and is located on a relatively flat area of the abdomen away from scars, dips and bends. It protrudes enough from the abdomen (one-half to one inch, 13–25 mm) to serve as a spout directing stool or urine into a pouch.

Often the stoma for a temporary ostomy doesn't meet these criteria. Frequently the patient can't tolerate more surgery and/or the surgeon may expend little time on a "temporary" measure. Too, it's often located in the transverse colon, near or above the waistline, which can be a difficult location for pouch and skin care later. If it's a loop ostomy, it may be quite large.

For a single end stoma in the ileum or in the first two-thirds of the colon, one uses the standard pouching techniques for an ileostomy. This means a drainable pouch with a bottom that can be opened, a skin barrier worn between pouch and skin to protect the skin from stool enzymes, and meticulous skin care. (See *Chapter 12— Pouches and the Skin They Touch* and *Chapter 13— Pouch Skills*.)

Although many of these are colostomies, they use part of the colon (often the transverse colon) in which the stool is still quite loose, like the stool in an ileostomy. The feces has gone only part of the way in its journey through the digestive tract and still contains a considerable amount of water. This loose feces pools on any exposed skin, and the normal stool enzymes begin digesting the skin just as they would any food.

(Sometimes the temporary end colostomy occurs in the descending or sigmoid colon, and it eventually passes formed stool. If so, and if this is a rather long-term ostomy, some people prefer to manage it with irrigation, a regularly-scheduled enema through the stoma so that stool passes at the person's convenience and not at other times. See Chapter 9—*Permanent Colostomies: Changes and Choices*.)

If there's a mucous fistula not too close to the stoma, it can be treated separately, with just a gauze square or other light covering to protect it and to protect clothing from any mucus. If stoma and mucous fistula are close, they can share one drainable pouch with a large stoma opening. (This is more difficult to care for and, fortunately, most surgeons usually don't place the stoma next to the mucous fistula.) A wafer of skin barrier can be cut with the two openings or an oval opening can be cut in the skin barrier to accommodate both stomas, with the area between the stomas filled with skin barrier paste. In any event, all the area around the stoma must be protected with some kind of skin barrier so that the stool enzymes don't get access to the skin.

For a loop ostomy, some manufacturers make a special pouch set which includes a large wafer of skin barrier (loop ostomies may be several inches or centimeters in diameter), a pouch with a large opening, and a rod to fit under the loop. If the surgeon uses the rod during the operation, it stays in place for several days and then is removed. The rod may have ends that can be flipped up or swiveled to make pouch application easier.

Otherwise, if there's a rod in place, a wafer of skin barrier can be cut to fit the stoma and then a straight cut can be made from the top edge down to the stoma opening. The prepared wafer is then applied around the stoma under the rod, with the cut ends brought together at the top of the stoma, away from the direction the stoma drains. Once the rod (if any) is removed, skin barrier preparation and pouch application are the same as for any stoma.

Ostomies with an inserted tube (cecostomies or nephrosotomies, for instance) drain through the tube into a collecting bag. If there's any leakage around the tube, the skin needs skin barrier protection. An alternative is to let the tube drain into a regular ostomy pouch adhered to the skin.

Temporary urostomies without a tube can usually be managed with a correctly-fitted pouch and a skin barrier to protect all the area around the stoma. Small pediatric pouches fit the little patients with temporary ostomies.

Of course, some temporary ostomies behave beautifully. There's never a whisper of a problem and the skin stays perfectly healthy. But in case of any problem, it's worth traveling a long way, if necessary, to get help from an ET nurse. The ET nurse can give individual guidance

Pouching a double-barrel ostomy
with stomas close together

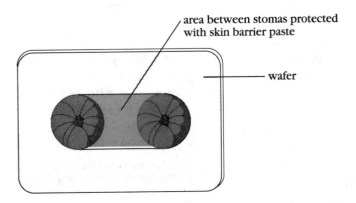

area between stomas protected
with skin barrier paste

wafer

about such things as managing the pouch at the waistline
that pulls loose when one bends (a belt and cement,
perhaps, or a nonadhesive pouch).

Why spend so much time and effort on skin care for
something that's supposed to last for only a short time?
It's worth it to keep comfortable; irritated skin hurts. Also
pouches don't adhere well to raw, roughened skin, so
there are more leaks and the problem gets worse. (That
also means more time is spent changing pouches.) Injured
skin means odor and possible infection. Sometimes the
skin is damaged permanently, which makes any reconnection surgery far more difficult.

(Most of the time, reconnection of a temporary ostomy
is a fairly simple surgery. The loop ostomy is stitched back
together and dropped back into the abdomen, or the
stoma and the mucous fistula (or Hartmann pouch) are
reconnected. Bowel preparation is similar to that required
before non-emergency ostomy surgery, except that irrigations or enemas may be necessary through stoma, mucous
fistula and/or anus, depending on the type of ostomy.

Pouching a loop ostomy
with attached rod

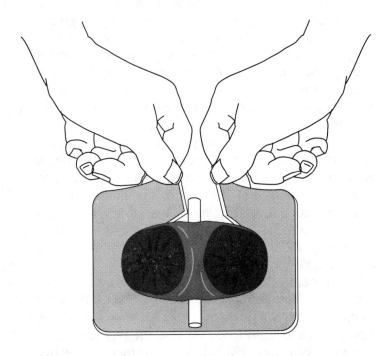

Surprisingly, living *without* pouches and passing stool
"normally" again through the anal sphincters may take a
period of adjustment.)

If skin care is important with a temporary ostomy, mind
care is even more so. Some people have little trouble
living with a temporary ostomy; others find it difficult to
make any "commitment" at all to a change that is supposed
to be short-term. Some people may believe that a temporary ostomy doesn't merit the emotional investment of
grief or anger; others find it hard to justify getting practical
help from an ET nurse or moral support from the United
Ostomy Association. Indeed, there is no one right way to
deal with a temporary ostomy, but there are ways of

thinking about and living with a temporary ostomy that many people have found helpful.

It takes time for anyone to adjust to this startling change in personal plumbing. And there's a tendency, when the ostomy is a temporary one, to resist even beginning to accept the change. Perhaps it seems that by accepting the ostomy, one somehow makes it more permanent. By not accepting the ostomy as "part of me," maybe one can get rid of it sooner. (This doesn't make sense, of course, but then, feelings and fears aren't particularly sensible.)

For a few days after surgery, many people ignore the stoma entirely (or just take a quick peek), while nurses perform any care. This is partly weakness, pain and anesthesia "hangover," and partly the human being's natural wisdom in confronting change slowly, denying it for a time. Also, as part of the quiet time, the digestive tract is also resting. (Urinary tract stomas start putting out urine immediately).

When the digestive tract wakes up, it does so with a vengeance. Most ostomies are on their worst behavior then, and then calm down over the next weeks. Suddenly there's much to learn to do. At first, the physical details of ostomy care seem overwhelming. If there's a change in self-image, it's probably to "an ostomy which happens to have a person attached"!

It's easy for the person with a new temporary ostomy to get stuck in the "ignore it and maybe it will go away" phase. It's equally easy to get so involved in physical care of the stoma and the skin around it that one can keep painful feelings at bay.

But those painful feelings are there, acknowledged or not. Indeed, it is outrageous that this happened. And sad. It's natural to be angry and human to grieve. Temporary or not, this is a major (and often unwelcome) change. Many people feel as if they are on an emotional roller coaster. (The physical demands of recovery from surgery and whatever led to it magnify these feelings.)

Sometimes, people—either the person with the ostomy or the people around—downplay the need for grieving about a "temporary" change. But this process of mourning seems to be necessary: Tears launder the soul. (See *Chapter 7—But How Do You Really Feel?*)

This all takes time. If the ostomy is for only a few weeks, there may not be time to get past the earliest stages. But even if it's very short term, it's worth coming to reconnection surgery with skin in good shape, time well-spent between surgeries, and the knowledge that one has coped well with a difficult situation. Life is too short to put "on hold."

Sometimes, too, temporary ostomies last longer than expected. Michael, for instance, went back for an internal reservoir surgery three months after his colon was removed for ulcerative colitis. The surgeon (one of the best) tried but couldn't make the reservoir; he held out hope that it might be possible "later." That was two years ago. Michael's "temporary" ostomy is still with him and, although he's healthy and back at work, he admits rather sheepishly that parts of his life are still "on hold."

How does one deal with a temporary ostomy? First, no matter how long the ostomy is supposed to last, it's smart to learn well how to care for the skin around the stoma and how to apply a pouch which stays on. This minimizes discomfort, time spent, and hassles—and means one can get on with living. An ET nurse or a knowledgeable hospital or home health nurse is the resource.

It's essential to find out enough about this particular ostomy to protect oneself from problems. For instance, if the stool is liquid and copious, it's important to know how much and what to drink. (If stool is liquid, see *Chapter 10—Ileostomies.*) If there are two openings in one stoma or two stomas present, it helps to know which one discharges stool and which is the mucous fistula.

Learning how to care for oneself (if that's physically possible) means gaining a measure of control over what's happening. Applying a pouch which stays on securely, learning a skin care skill, knowing what to do to prevent noise, odor or "bag bulge" all give a person mastery over a difficult new situation. That is satisfying. (Accidents may happen; that's part of the learning process and occasionally inevitable with even the most experienced care.)

But pouching techniques aren't the hardest skill to acquire with a temporary ostomy. It's much more difficult to learn how to take one day at a time, to enjoy the journey instead of just waiting for the destination. Looking forward to eventual reconnection, of course. That's only human. But to defer everything until *after* can be a massive waste of time.

With a secure pouch, it's time to get healthy again, which means eating well, walking or exercising as the doctor allows, laughing, doing enjoyable things. Thinking more about living, and less about ill health or pouches. Work or travel may be possible, or this may be time for learning a new skill or indulging in a hobby.

Like any crisis, this one offers a chance for reassessing priorities, appreciating what is good, and looking toward necessary changes. A temporary ostomy can be perceived as either an intolerable disaster, or as a challenge and an opportunity for personal growth.

For instance, learning to care for the skin around the stoma is a chance to take care of oneself. Drawing on personal strengths to cope with this change can make people appreciate their ability to survive the difficult and unfamiliar. (Of course, it also means being gentle and forgiving with oneself, because not everything will go smoothly.) And it's definitely a time to laugh, sometimes to keep from crying, or just because it's all rather ridiculous.

This is also a time for letting other people help, usually

not so much with the physical care of the ostomy as with emotional support (or a good meal or just being there). Some family members and friends are splendid—but others don't seem able to cope, perhaps because this is so new to them, perhaps for other reasons. (An ET nurse may be able to help in some cases.) In fact, many people tend to be wonderfully supportive at times and less so at others. Sometimes they're dealing with their own varying emotions, or sometimes they find that the person with the ostomy acts differently from one day to the next.

Calling on the local United Ostomy Association for an ostomy visitor can be helpful. (One tip: Many temporary colostomies act a lot more like ileostomies than like permanent colostomies so that an ostomy visitor with an ileostomy may be able to help, if no one who has had a temporary ostomy is available.) UOA chapters can also provide "family visitors" (such as a spouse who can talk with the patient's spouse). ET nurses or doctors may have names of other possible visitors.

No one has to be enthusiastic about an ostomy, temporary or permanent. What is required is reasonable care. What is *hoped* for is a beginning acceptance of the ostomy as "part of me"—a temporary slight change in the plumbing, that is a small price to pay for life, health and well-being.

CHAPTER 15 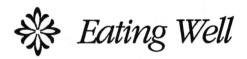 *Eating Well*

> . . .*she opened it, and found in it a very small*
> *cake, on which the words, "EAT ME" were*
> *beautifully marked in currants. "Well, I'll eat it",*
> *said Alice, "and if it makes me larger, I can*
> *reach the key; and if it makes me smaller,*
> *I can creep under the door.* . . .
> Lewis Carroll, *Alice in Wonderland*

"Curiouser and curiouser," cried Alice—and people with ostomies, confused about what they can and should eat, might well echo the bewildered lass. Someone says, "Eat what your doctor says." But then the doctor says, "Eat what you want." What to do?

If the person with a new ostomy is perplexed, trying to juggle protein and "residue" and electrolytes and calories and dollars, he's not alone. "The only thing I can count on now," said a friend of ours who doesn't have an ostomy, "is that if I like some food, an expert will say 'It's bad for you'!" Or it costs too much.

In the midst of this muddle, a few points remain clear. Everyone, with or without an ostomy needs to be well nourished. Surgery hasn't changed the physical (or the emotional) need for good food.

For the first week or two after ostomy surgery, the

question of what's for dinner tomorrow remains academic, and more than a little dull. Until the digestive tract settles down, the patient is stuck with bland, easily-digested food. Then, as the sense of adventure regenerates, the longing for greener pastures—or at least a leaf of lettuce—returns. Fortunately, the greener pastures are usually within reach. Most people, after they recuperate, can eat most foods.

Eating well is one of the real rewards for the person who has undergone ileostomy surgery for inflammatory bowel disease, and who has been banished to boiled rice and applesauce too long. Whenever cancer is involved (as it often is with colostomies and urostomies), eating well is one of the best kinds of medicine, for both body and spirit. And, whatever the major surgery, food's the real lifeline for getting the body strong and fit again.

First things first: How do we become well nourished?

The body needs raw materials for the processes necessary for life—and it needs a steady source of them. Food supplies these building blocks for energy and for tissue growth and repair in the body. It also provides some of the chemical regulators which the body needs to change these raw materials into energy and tissue. To do all this, the body needs six different kinds of *nutrients*, or specific components of food: carbohydrates, proteins, fats, vitamins, minerals, and water.

Most foods combine all or several of these components. Milk, for instance, contains all six (including some of the vitamins and minerals, although not all). So does a cucumber, but the amounts are less, and the proportions are different. Putting foods together so that we get enough of each nutrient to keep the body operating—and there are endless ways to do this—is how we nourish ourselves. Thanks to the variety, we can add foods we like, subtract those we can't afford, substitute intelligently (grains, nuts, milk, and eggs for meat, for example), and still emerge with healthy, delicious, affordable fare.

A few years ago, nutritionists figured out a fairly simple way for people to put together a healthy, well-balanced diet without having to count each gram of carbohydrate, every milligram of vitamin B_2. If adults eat or drink two 8-ounce servings of milk (or the equivalent in milk products), two 3-ounce servings of meat or high protein foods (fish, eggs, nuts, soybeans, for instance), four helpings of fruit or vegetables (1/2 cup cooked vegetable or one fresh orange is one serving), and four servings of cereal and grains (one slice of bread equals one serving) each day, they probably get the basic nutrients they need.

There's a move now toward reducing the amount of animal protein and fat in the diet and increasing the grains, fruits and vegetables. Many people work out their meals around combinations of lower protein non-animal foods which, eaten together, give the body the nutrients it needs.

Some people with ostomies have special needs for three of the nutrients: vitamins, minerals, and water.

Many nutritionists believe that a healthy, varied selection of foods provides all the vitamins (the chemical regulators the body needs in tiny amounts to keep running smoothly) most people need. There is one exception for some of those whose ostomy surgery involves the very end of the ileum: vitamin B_{12}, which is absorbed in the section of intestine where small and large bowel join. Even when all of this ileal segment is removed during surgery, many people seem to have little trouble, but some may need a B_{12} injection every few months. Loss of appetite and decreased energy may result from a deficiency; a check with the doctor is in order.

Electrolyte is a common term in ostomy language. An electrolyte is an electrical charge which plays a big role in how the body functions. These charges come from minerals (such as sodium, potassium and calcium) dissolved in the body fluids.

When all or most of the large intestine, which absorbs

some electrolytes and about one-tenth of the water needed by the body, is missing, the nonabsorbed water and electrolytes are released in liquid or soft stool. Potassium and other electrolytes sometimes wash out faster than the body can replenish them. Potassium-rich foods, like bananas, oranges, prunes, and tomatoes (and there are many more; lists are readily available), solve the problem most of the time. Potassium also comes as a liquid or powder supplement, to be used with medical supervision only.

Sodium tends to be less of a problem, since the typical American diet contains far more salt than the body can use, but most people who have loose stools from an ostomy can use a little extra salt. During a short bout of diarrhea or vomiting, or during very hot weather, they can replace unusual losses with an electrolyte-rich "sports" drink or a homemade recipe. (One calls for 1 teaspoon each salt and baking soda, 4 teaspoons white corn syrup, and one 6-ounce can frozen orange juice in enough water to make 1 quart—1/2 cup to be drunk every hour.) If the problem continues, medical help is essential.

People don't think of water as food, but it, too, is an essential nutrient, needed in constant supply. With the short-circuit in their water-absorbing colon, those with loose stools require even more water, and food with large water content, than most people do; the kidneys, which do most of the regulating of water and electrolytes in the body, compensate for some of the loss. Drinking more water does *not* increase bowel output because most of the water is absorbed by the small intestine. People with ileostomies need to keep drinking so that the substances that cause kidney stones and gallstones keep flushing out of the kidneys. Those who have urostomies also need to keep drinking so that any bacteria that may cause kidney infection keep washing out of the conduit.

Many Americans—with and without ostomies—worry

about their weight. Everyone has a favorite diet, whether it's a bedraggled carrot and lettuce leaf smorgasbord or a melon mania. For the person with an ileostomy, especially, the problem may sneak up. Before surgery, gaining each pound was a desperate struggle; suddenly, after surgery, bulges and double-chins appear. Others may be trying to gain weight, and they too will be counting *calories*, those measures of heat (energy) released when a food is processed in the body. (3500 calories beyond what the body needs to maintain itself means one pound of extra weight; this extra fat comes from carbohydrates, fats, protein, and alcohol.)

The common-sense approach to dieting starts with making food really *work* in the body. Most foods contain several of the six nutrient types, so that they are doing other things for the body *besides* creating calories of energy. The "junk foods," on the other hand—the candy, the cookies from refined sugar, the alcohol—provide calories and that's about all. We still have to eat all the rest of the foods, which incidentally also contain calories, to meet our bodies' needs.

Most nutritionists agree that although the body needs fats, it doesn't need nearly as many of them as the typical diet includes. Since fats are concentrated sources of calories, they are a leverage food for losing or gaining weight.

Fiber—also called roughage or residue or bulk—is a recent darling of the nutritionists. Fiber is an undigestible carbohydrate (like bran and parts of fruits and vegetables). It contributes nothing to human nutrition, but acts as a sponge in the intestine, soaking up water to soften the stool and speed it on its way. Fiber can be either water-soluble or water-insoluble. The water-soluble kind, found in fruits, oat bran, barley and legumes (like beans), breaks down somewhat in the body's digestive juices to form a gummy substance which can lower blood cholesterol levels. The other kind, found in vegetables, wheat and bran (except oat bran) cereals, doesn't break down at all; it seems to help protect the body against some cancers, including colon cancer.

In general, a low-residue diet tends to be constipating, while a high-fiber diet leads to looser, more frequent stools. It can take the body a while to adapt to more bulk, so it should be introduced slowly into the diet.

Those with colostomies can balance the amount of fiber in their diets (along with the amounts of fluids and exercise) so that they have a soft, formed stool which passes easily. On the other hand, the digestive tracts of most people with ileostomies can't handle a very high-fiber diet, laced with large quantities of bran.

Many people do very nicely by avoiding both extremes and aiming for moderate residue, with some whole grain breads and cereals, and some raw or partially cooked fruits and vegetables. The person with an ileostomy may tolerate this amount of bulk with ease, or may be willing to cope with more frequent emptying of a pouch.

Most people with ostomies can eat most things. But it's an individual matter. Considering how important eating well is, it would be great if there were ileostomy diets, colostomy diets, and urostomy diets, all ready to hand out along with any other hospital discharge material. Unfortunately, there's a lot more trial and error than that.

One woman, from Coos Bay, Oregon, reported: "When I had my ileostomy, my surgeon told me I could eat anything that agreed with me. After so many years of diet because of ulcerative colitis, I could hardly believe my ears! However, that little phrase, 'that agreed with me,' was the joker."

She checked with others and found that everyone had a few foods to avoid—but they were different foods for different individuals: "One eats applesauce to stop the 'runs' while I eat applesauce if I need something to act as a mild laxative."

"Our systems are so different, no one, not even a doctor, can give you a diet list and expect it to work for you. . . as for an ileostomy diet, there is no such thing! We find out, sometimes the hard way, if we have eaten something we shouldn't."

It's best to go slowly after surgery, adding a small amount of a new food at a time and then waiting 24–48 hours to see what happens. Even if a food disagrees the first time, it can be tried again a few weeks later, perhaps in a smaller amount. And if peanuts don't work, maybe peanut butter will. The blender can make foods that are too fibrous more tolerable.

Many people with ileostomies and a few with colostomies avoid, or eat sparingly, foods with a large amount of *cellulose*, a kind of fiber found in popcorn, coconut, stringy celery, shells of peas, and such Chinese vegetables as bean sprouts and bamboo shoots. These, along with granola-type cereals and nuts, especially when taken in large amounts, and hastily chewed, are the villains in most food blockages (obstructions). In a *blockage*, the bowel clogs up with undigested food, the ostomy stops functioning, and the abdomen starts cramping. (Since it's made from the small intestine, an ileostomy is much more at risk for obstruction from food than a colostomy, which has a larger diameter.)

Most blockages resolve themselves quickly. First step is to put on a disposable appliance with a large stoma opening, so that the swelling stoma is not constricted. Then, simple remedies can be tried, like changing position or relaxing in the bath. (If the ostomy doesn't start working again after two hours or so, it's time for medical help.)

There'd be far fewer blockages if all people with ostomies were better chewers, but. . .One of the food Messiahs around the turn of the century was a gentleman named Fletcher, who tried to sell "Fletcherism": chewing every bite of food 30 times. Probably the person who revived Fletcherism could eat anything. On the other hand, such a safe and cautious approach might spoil the fun for people like our friend Rachel, who occasionally delights in calling a dish of popcorn and a glass of lemonade lunch, just to prove she can!

People with ileostomies or colostomies have no monopoly on passing gas. But they probably worry about it more because it comes through the abdomen—and involuntarily—rather than through the rectum, and more voluntarily. Too, gas in a pouch makes it bulge.

The cause and the solution can vary. Digestive tracts seem to work most efficiently with meals at regular times, although this may mean three times a day, or several smaller meals. Skipping a meal invites increased gas.

Swallowed air can work its way through the digestive tract to be expelled as gas. Eating slowly, sipping rather than gulping drinks, giving up chewing gum, not talking while eating, all can reduce air swallowing. With their built-in bubbles, carbonated drinks (like sodas and beer) are notorious gas-causers.

The digestive tract works on some foods (including onions, cabbage, baked beans, cucumbers, turnips and radishes) to produce gas for many people, with or without ostomies. Too, many adults no longer produce lactase, the enzyme which breaks down the lactose in dairy products; if they drink or eat milk products, this *lactose intolerance* gives them cramping and gas. Cutting out or cutting down on dairy products is one solution. Another possibility is using reduced-lactose dairy products from the grocery store, or lactase enzyme pills or drops from the pharmacy.

To resolve major problems with gas, a little detective work may be in order, along with a willingness to give up a problem food. Observing when gas occurs, and remembering what was eaten in the last several hours, provide the clues. In the meantime, many people swear by their favorite dietary remedies for gas and the odor from it: parsley, tomato juice, or buttermilk perhaps, or yogurt (preferably the plain variety, with active cultures/enzymes, flavored with fresh fruits at home.)

If the offender is the "trapped gas" dear to TV commercials, anything which hastens peristalsis will hasten relief. A small meal, half a cup of coffee, exercise, or massaging the abdomen may help. Some use over-the-counter nostrums, but it's wise to consult a doctor before trying this.

Today's pouches are odor-proof. However, a bit of privacy when the gas is released may be comforting, since gas may have a strong odor. Gas can be dispersed out a special valve or through the bottom of a drainable pouch, or it can be "burped" out the top of some two-piece pouches. A much less desirable option is poking a pinhole in a pouch to release gas and then patching the hole with non-porous tape; this breaks the integrity of the odor-proof pouch. For many people who irrigate, irrigation and some attention to diet can be enough to keep the person as free from gas and odor as any human being can be; otherwise, a small pouch suffices.

Some people have special diet needs. Free booklets on eating well during cancer treatment can be ordered through the Cancer Information Service of the National Cancer Institute (1-800-4-CANCER). The book *Nutrition for the Chemotherapy Patient*, by Ramstack and Rosenbaum (Bull Publishing Co., 1990) has concrete suggestions for the person undergoing chemotherapy.

People with ostomies who form kidney stones or gallstones need guidance from a doctor or dietitian on what foods to avoid. Those with other medical problems, such as high blood pressure or diabetes, can learn about their particular diets with the help of a dietitian.

The U.S. Government publishes a wealth of free or low-cost brochures and booklets about nutrition, meal planning, thrifty recipes, and similar topics. A postcard to the Consumer Information Center, Pueblo, Colorado 81009, will bring a complete list of publications.

Our bodies depend on good food. Our spirits, no less, are nourished, whether by the hearty stew shared with family, the romantic candle-lit dinner with a loved one, or the meal prepared with care by the person living alone, and served with a vase of daisies on the tray.

Food is an adventure, and a delight. From time to time, it's even worth breaking a rule or two. That's how our friend Ann feels about it. Says Ann, who has had her ileostomy for many years: "I love cucumbers, always have. They bring back summer. . . and picnics when I was a kid. Sure, I know that cucumbers don't like me much, that I'll be emptying my appliance all the time if I eat one.

"But every once in a while. . .it's worth it!"

CHAPTER 16   ❀   *Catnaps,*
Strolls, and Good Belly
Laughs

It's time to go, to run, to rise up, to fling open the
window, thaw the blood, prance high in the wet
grass—to shout and feel and seek new rootholds
in the nourishing earth.
William Hedgepeth

When Neanderthal Ned ventured out of his cave some
thousands of years ago—and found himself face-to-face
with a large and furious beast—his body responded. Ned's
adrenals, tiny glands nestled above each kidney, sent an
instant chemical message to the rest of the body: Emergency! Ned's heart raced, pumping blood laced with
oxygen through ready vessels to lungs, arms, legs, shunt-
ing it away from the rest of the body during this crisis. If
the beast was very large, and maybe a little slow and
nearsighted, Ned took to his heels, fleeing danger. Or,
strength surging, Ned faced and fought the beast. The
crisis resolved quickly. Sometimes Ned won, sometimes
the beast.

Modern man lives in different circumstances—with the same body. Evolving over millions of years to survive short emergencies, the body has not progressed (or regressed) to fit the way many of us live now. Faced with any kind of change in its equilibrium, it reacts in the same all-out fashion: Blood vessels constrict, heart pounds, skin perspires to cope with the increased heat of racing blood, digestive tract slows to a halt, sexual energies dissolve. This generalized body reaction is called stress; whatever evokes the reaction (such as an attacking beast) is called a stressor.

But, except for the rare emergency (like grabbing a child out of the path of an onrushing car), we usually face chronic rather than acute stressors. And often we can neither fight nor flee. Instead we continue to face the same stressful situations day after day, month after month: a demanding job, a difficult (and unchangeable) employer, daily traffic jams, inflation, illness, worries about those dear to us. All too often we can neither resolve the problem nor get away from it.

Hans Selye, a Canadian physiologist who accidentally discovered what happened to adrenal glands under continuing stress, led the way to a whole new perspective on health and illness. He considers stress "the spice of life," a good and necessary thing in our lives—within reason. We cannot change or grow without stress: "Since stress is associated with all types of activity, we could avoid most of it only by never doing anything. Who would enjoy a life of no runs, no hits, no errors!"

But constant stress becomes *distress* and does peculiar and devastating things to the body. Blood vessels, constricted by adrenalin, forget how to relax, perhaps leading to high blood pressure. With the action shunted away from it to the emergency centers of the body, the digestive tract slows down—and a multi-million-dollar laxative industry springs up.

And the poor adrenals, expected to cope with never-ending crises, grow weary. Increasingly-sturdy research points to a connection between serious disease and grinding chronic stress. Our bodies deal successfully every day with disease-causers: bacteria, viruses, carcinogens (cancer-causing substances). If our defenses are strong, we don't get sick as easily. But, with unremitting stress, the body's protective systems grow exhausted or confused. Invaders slip past—bringing perhaps just a cold, perhaps cancer. Or the body starts seeing invaders where there aren't any and begins attacking itself, as may happen in inflammatory bowel disease.

If we get the message, along with our ostomy surgery, either that we've been facing too many stressors, or that our system for coping with them needs an overhaul, we can seize the chance to become healthier and happier than we've ever been. (Obviously, the disease, the surgery and the new ostomy add to the pressure temporarily.) Knowing there's a problem is the first step toward solving it.

When our friend Helen was recovering from throat cancer, for example, her doctor insisted that she cut down the stress in her life. That's a tall order, but Helen took it seriously. She simplified here, and delegated authority there. She described to us one change—small, but telling: As a bit of "self-discipline," she had gotten into the habit of always swallowing the large number of pills prescribed for her *before* yielding to the demands of her bladder, however urgent. Now the bladder wins!

If we listen to them, our bodies can often tell us things we wouldn't dare to admit to ourselves. Kathy, who doesn't have an ostomy, confesses: "I always knew I didn't like my boss—but I didn't realize *how* furious I was at him. Finally I put two and two together and figured out that the only time my bowel wasn't on the warpath was when he was sick or on vacation—then I knew I had to make a change."

Many of those with ostomies could echo her. Since the digestive tract (and even the urinary tract, sometimes) turns sluggish or starts racing partly in response to the stress messages of the body, our ostomies warn us that maybe some quiet moments are overdue. How relaxed we are certainly isn't the only factor in making an ostomy behave happily—but it's a *big* one.

Some stressors we can't avoid. But some we can. The Serenity Prayer (page 50)—changing what can be changed, accepting what can't be changed, and knowing the difference—says it best. Often, if we can *space* or *postpone* the avoidable stressors, we can manage the unavoidable ones. We also may be able to change the way that we *perceive* stressors so that they lose their power to distress us. For instance, we might mentally "re-frame" a long, tense daily commute into an opportunity to think quietly, or to listen to enjoyable music or a book on tape.

Sometimes we need help. For comfort and reassurance as we encounter unavoidable stressors, family, friends, doctor, and clergymen can lend a hand. Sometimes, with personal counseling, we learn that we are putting ourselves under intolerable pressure to maintain a particular image of ourselves. When we can let go of that "Superman" or "Perfect Mother" (or whatever) image, we find out that we *can* avoid some of those "unavoidable" stressors. And if we can let go the burdens of yesterday and tomorrow, we are free to enjoy the pleasures of today.

Neanderthal Ned faced his share of stress. But if he survived the encounter with large-and-furious beast, he had a chance to loll about the cave a bit, chew a few berries, and have a pleasant dinner of ex-furious beast. Even if we can't change our stressor load, we can give our bodies a chance to rest up, to recuperate from the arrows of daily life.

When Norman Cousins, then editor of *The Saturday Review*, heard his acute illness diagnosed as a life-threatening disease in 1964, he searched back over the past hectic

Catnaps, Strolls, and Good Belly Laughs   175

months for possible causes. It became more and more clear to him that an exhausted adrenal system, worn out by both acute and chronic stress without relief, was a big factor. Since there was no known treatment for the disease, Cousins decided, with his doctor's encouragement, to bolster the tired adrenals, using his own therapy of belly laughs and vitamin C. Comedy film clips and anthologies of humor took the place of pain shots. As he tells it in *Anatomy of an Illness* (Norton, 1979), he "made the joyous discovery that ten minutes of genuine belly laughter had an anesthetic effect and would give me at least two hours of pain-free sleep." The disease retreated.

Exercise is another natural relaxer. In fact, since our body's stress response equips it to flee or to fight, running—or walking, or in fact any vigorous activity—is ideal. It's what our body wants us to do. A brisk walk around the block clears not only the mind but the body.

Slow deep breathing, too, holds a special magic. As part of exercise, or on its own, it gets rid of some of the chemical residue of the body's stress response. And it feels so good. Taking slow deep breaths, we fill the lungs. It's an ancient technique for relaxing, cheaper and safer than tranquilizers or alcohol.

Sometimes we have a hobby or favorite activity that lets the tension slip away like an ebbing tide. As we pick up a trowel in the garden, or sit down at the piano, or take a stitch in the embroidery, we can feel a gentle relaxation flow over us. Doing something for ourselves, whether it's listening to a favorite piece of music or reading a good book or talking to a friend, revives us. Or maybe it's just doing something completely different from our usual job—perhaps working at a hospital as a volunteer once a week—that recharges us.

People we care about and who care about us can be a major buffer against stress. These social contacts can be family and friends, or perhaps members of a church, interest group, or support group (UOA or a cancer support group, maybe). Being around caring people just seems to ease the load.

And then there's sleep. "That we are not much sicker and much madder than we are," writes Aldous Huxley, "is due exclusively to that most blessed and blessing of all natural graces, sleep."

Whether it's a catnap or a full eight hours, sleep refreshes. Sleep restores. And how well we sleep is also a subtle barometer of how well we are dealing with the stressors in our lives.

Perhaps Neanderthal Ned slipped into sleep as effortlessly as a kitten does. But with our different kind of pressures, we don't always sleep soundly and easily. Surgery can be a springboard for dependence on sleeping pills; it's easy, and sometimes necessary, to resort to this chemical aid in the hospital when pain, unfamiliar surroundings, hospital noise, lack of exercise, and anxiety take their toll. But over long periods, sleeping pills don't work well.

There are better answers. Some gentle exercise before bedtime, a warm bath, a good (but not too exciting) book, a glass of warm milk, are all natural soporifics, lulling us to natural sleep. A bedtime routine (even without the teddy bear tuck-in!) readies us. A comfortable bed helps.

But the core of the matter is relaxation. No matter how comfortable the bed, no matter how tired we are, there is no way for us to sleep peacefully with taut muscles, clenched jaws and a racing mind. Luckily, we can learn how to relax; it's a skill we can draw on during the day as well as at bedtime.

Many people find one of the meditation techniques effective. By concentrating on one word or phrase for a time, at regular intervals, they slip into serene relaxation. Picturing an appealing scene (perhaps a secluded, sun-drenched beach) relaxes others. Some people find that praying—laying troubles in the lap of a higher being—is all they need.

Or we can approach relaxation from another angle and relax the body physically. Although it may seem like putting the cart before the horse, the relaxed body seems to draw the mind with it.

One method for relaxing the body involves first tensing a small group of muscles (like the arm), becoming aware of just how it feels, and then slowly, consciously, releasing the tension, feeling it flow away. Starting with legs and arms and trunk, one works up to shoulders, neck, jaw. What surprises most of us when we're learning how to relax is finding out just how tense we are most of the time. It takes a while to learn how to unknot those muscles at will. There are some quick first-aid techniques for relaxing. Shaking an arm or leg, for instance, unkinks those taut muscles.

Relaxation classes, books on relaxing, stress reduction clinics, professional massage, sophisticated technology (like biofeedback, in which a person learning to relax hears a tone indicating how taut or relaxed a muscle is and gradually learns to sustain the "relaxed tone") all are ways of helping a tense world unwind.

Unless we're lumps, we face stressors in our lives. So probably we all could use some healthy way of handling those pressures. Some kind of relaxation belongs in our daily lives.

We each find our own ways. Nadine Stair wrote about her ways—at age 85:

"If I had to live my life over again, I'd dare to make more mistakes next time.

I'd relax.

I would limber up.

I would be sillier than I have been this trip.

I would take fewer things seriously.

I would take more chances.

I would take more trips. I would climb more mountains, swim more rivers.

I would eat more ice cream and less beans.

I would perhaps have more actual troubles, but I'd have fewer imaginary ones.

You see, I'm one of those people who live seriously and sanely hour after hour, day after day.

Oh, I've had my moments. And if I had it to do over again, I'd have more of them.

In fact, I'd try to have nothing else, just moments, one after another, instead of living so many years ahead of each day.

I've been one of those persons who never goes anywhere without a thermometer, a hot water bottle, a raincoat and a parachute.

If I had it to do again I would travel lighter than I have.

If I had to live my life over, I would start barefoot earlier in the spring, and stay that way later in fall.

I would go to more dances.

I would ride more merry-go-rounds.

I would pick more daisies."

CHAPTER 17　　　🏵️　　　*You're Looking Great!*

Beware of all enterprises that require new
clothes, and not rather a new wearer of clothes.
Henry David Thoreau

We are new wearers of clothes, given new life by a surgical detour. And while the enterprise may not *require* new clothes (except for maybe a bathing suit with a slightly different cut), an ostomy is a grand excuse for a little shopping.

In the beginning, shuffling down the hall in a baggy hospital gown, dragging a reluctant IV pole in my wake, I found it hard to believe I'd ever look really good again or be able to wear anything but shapeless sacks or rumpled bathrobes. In theory, especially after meeting a UOA visitor or two, smartly dressed in snug-fitting clothes, I knew it could be done. But! Incision tender, abdomen puffy, stoma still almost a stranger and covered with that unfamiliar post-op pouch, perineal wound draining and tweaking like a toothache, I felt uncomfortable, awkward, and unattractive. Looking great? Nonsense! As my mother used to say, I looked as if I were sent for and couldn't come.

It's a little like getting back to normal after having a baby. The woman who tries to wear her pre-pregnancy slacks home from the hospital after delivery finds it just doesn't work—at first. A few weeks later, they may fit fine.

As the incision healed, the stoma shrank, and pain became something I could barely remember, I began to notice clothing ads in the morning paper. And to remember how smart Ann and Dorothy looked. Person after person has reported disbelief—and the beginning of hope—when they met their first UOA visitor. Whatever else they forget, they all seem to remember that the visitor was well dressed! As one woman reported in the Metro Maryland newsletter, "In less than two hours, a lovely lady entered my room, beautifully dressed, and announced who she was. From that day on everything improved. Her image has been with me these past four years."

Clothes that look good and feel good are an important bridge back to the world, one way of mending a bruised body image and moving ahead from *patient* to *person*. A well-cut sports coat or a new haircut is a flag being raised with the message: "I'm not licked!"

An ostomy seldom limits anyone's clothing horizons; sometimes it expands them. As a result, people with an ostomy are perhaps a little better dressed than the average person. They've learned that looking good is important to their own morale, even if no one sees but the mirror. Looking good also brings positive feedback. I discovered that when a friend said, "Wow! You look great!" I felt better. And when—instead of offering sympathy or chicken soup—they said, "Let's go out to lunch," I was almost mended.

Few people are ready for modeling assignments the first few weeks or even months after ostomy surgery. (I never was, but that had nothing to do with surgery.) Abdominal tenderness and, if the rectum and anus were removed, a still sore perineal area make looser than usual clothes comfortable. For women, this may mean wraparound skirts instead of form-fitting pants, and A-line dresses or gaudy caftans instead of snug sheaths. Until one gets used to a changed body, overblouses or shirts worn outside pants offer welcome reassurance. In this period, until they're sure their new control systems don't leak, many people prefer prints or plaids to solid colors, so any small accident would go unnoticed.

Night gowns (or night shirts) may feel better than pajamas. For both men and women, suspenders may be more tolerable temporarily than belts. Both may wish to change underwear types, switching to underpants with elastic above or below the stoma rather than right on top of it. For underpants, cotton absorbs perspiration better than synthetic fabrics, yet need not look like great aunt Minnie's winter drawers. If there is a perineal wound still draining, sanitary mini-pads affixed to underpants may be used.

After convalescence, there are few limits. Pouches are now so slim they don't show under snug clothing (with the possible exception of thin, clinging jerseys). Light-weight girdles for women and supports for men are optional (unless the doctor orders them). Pantyhose, as is or with the legs cut off, gently flatten a pouch. Tight girdles or belts which rub the stoma should be avoided.

The person with a stoma at the belt line or above may need considerable ingenuity in choosing clothes. Men may pick suspenders, heavier shirts, concealing sweaters, overshirts or jumpsuits; women may prefer looser styles, overblouses, and the like. Many of those with stomas at the waistline wear belts with their pouches for extra security when bending.

Thanks to the new flexibility in fashion, there are usually enough variations in style in any season so that it's easy to find something that's good looking, comfortable and as fashionable as one cares to be. If one designer hasn't come up with just the right thing this season, someone else probably has.

For ideas on looking good with an ostomy, nothing beats attending the local UOA meeting (or, a little later, a regional or national conference). My first meeting astounded me. I guess I'd expected a roomful of gloomy Joes and grim Gerties, all feeling sorry for themselves. But I was wrong, and I remember clearly my first impression: "These *can't* be people with ostomies. They look too good...." Perhaps they weren't all fashion plates, but they cared about their appearance, and about grooming. They knew the image they presented to the world was important, not only personally, but to people with new ostomies and the world in general.

If the budget permits, ostomy surgery provides a fine excuse for getting something new and pleasing to wear. Those with new ileostomies may want to hold off major clothing purchases for a bit until weight stabilizes. Before surgery, the problem was keeping weight up; now everything tastes so good, it may be hard to keep the extra pounds off.

However therapeutic a new wardrobe may be, medical insurance doesn't pay for it. There are alternatives. If money is scarce, ingenuity needn't be. Changing a collar style, shortening sleeves, adding a little embroidery, converting a tired dress to a fresh new skirt—there may be more in the closet than we think. Another possibility is a visit to a local thrift shop or a garage sale.

With returning energy and more dependable bodies, people with ostomies may need new kinds of clothes to follow new paths: a jogging suit, a business-like dress after a promotion, drip-dry separates for travel, clothes for dancing or swimming or tennis. Or even a wedding dress.

Vicki Cunning of Irving, Texas, found herself not only enjoying new clothes after her surgery, but modeling them as part of her job: "Suddenly it was zero hour and we were dressed. And ready? Well, maybe not completely ready inside, but it was too late now! Lights! Music! Action! My first outfit had buttons down the front. I was shaking so hard when I got off the stage someone had to unbutton it. I seemed to get braver (they had told us that we would), because the more that I went on the easier it got. We danced rather than just walked up and down that runway! Me, with an ileostomy! I was a model!"

Children with ostomies don't need special clothes—just ones they like. Those who have surgery to control dribbling urine now can enjoy in a world without wet pants or diapers and are free to wear clothes they couldn't risk before, including Little League uniforms and ballet costumes. As for any children, easy-care, comfortable clothes are best for school and play, with something special for big occasions.

For thousands of people with ostomies, the prognosis is excellent. For some, it's not that good. Our friend Trudy taught us that even a somewhat gloomy diagnosis is no reason to wear dreary clothes. During radiation and after, she lost a lot of weight. She'd always been proud of her figure and found her new scrawniness depressing, so she went shopping. In addition to an apricot plush housecoat that caught her eye, she got some soft cotton blouses with full sleeves, a skirt with a little more fullness, a jumper cut wide enough so she could wear turtlenecks under it, and a couple of gaudy kimonos.

"The new clothes weren't an extravagance, really. Wearing them, I feel better about myself and it's surprising how often friends say, 'You're looking great! ' They've stopped treating me like a thin china cup, and I'm enjoying each day more."

Among people with ostomies, some favor soft worn jeans, some are never caught in anything but the latest fashion, and there are thousands and thousands in between. In one way or another, though, clothes are a useful shorthand, telling the world, "An ostomy is OK—and so am I!"

CHAPTER 18 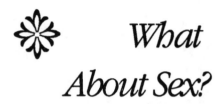 *What About Sex?*

> *Some things are better than sex, and some are*
> *worse, but there's nothing exactly like it.*
> W.C. Fields

From birth to death, we are sexual persons—and ostomy surgery doesn't change that. So it's natural to wonder about sex after surgery: "Can I?" "Will anyone want me?" "Can I enjoy it? Can I satisfy my partner and myself?"

For many people, sex can be as good as it was before, or even better (if surgery follows years of severe ulcerative colitis, for instance). People with ostomies date, fall in love, marry and have children. For some, there may be problems, temporary or permanent; even then, there are possible remedies and alternatives.

We bring all of ourselves to sex—our beliefs, expectations and experiences. Whether it's part of a loving long-term relationship or a shorter exploration, sex is a special kind of communication, one way of giving and receiving pleasure.

We bring our bodies to sex. Even more importantly, we bring our minds and emotions. The most important sex organ is not the penis or the clitoris, but the brain. That's where most difficulties with sex start—and where they can be solved. Neither bedroom acrobatics nor the titillations from the most exotic sex manual can compensate for severe anxiety, depression, exhaustion, or unwillingness or inability to talk to each other. But the mind, given a chance, can help.

About the time the abdominal incision heals (not many weeks after ostomy surgery, barring complications), the doctor will agree that the person can safely participate in the sex act. Before that, of course, caressing, stroking, touching, laughing, cuddling and all the other ways of showing love and caring are fine.

What sometimes happens, the first time, is a scenario like this: Jim, who recently underwent ileostomy surgery, decides that today's the day for the first lovemaking since surgery. If he'll admit it, he's still pretty tired; he doesn't realize how exhausting major abdominal surgery is. Too, he's feeling low, worried about things like money, getting back to work, and problems he can't quite put his finger on. Never mind. He's eager for some great sex. Still, he's a bit anxious. How will it go? What if his pouch slips? What if there's some odor? What if. . .? To calm his fears, he downs a couple of stiff drinks, climbs into bed. Disaster. He can't get an erection. The more he tries, the more frustrated he becomes. Angry and fearful, Jim blames his new ostomy. His wife consoles him—but she wonders too.

It's a classic scene. One surgeon lists four normal (and solvable) problems after surgery: "(a) Failure [of erection or orgasm] because of trying intercourse before strength returns following surgery. (b) Serious anxiety or fear of the ability to perform sexually, the attractiveness of one's altered body, the possibility of odor and the security of the appliance or stoma covering. (c) Depression which many people suffer following any surgery. (d) Excessive medication and/or alcohol."

A different scenario is possible for Jim. The next time around, he's a little more rested, he's begun to get some exercise again and to eat well. He's shed a few tears and lost his initial embarrassment. The big difference, though, is that Jim has been talking to his wife, Susan, really talking, and she's been talking too. That old myth of the male as the strong silent type without tears or doubts is just that—a myth. Reality, with men who are not afraid to feel and to talk about what they feel, is better.

Susan has her own worries and resentments. Some fears and angry feelings they can lay to rest. The others they can work on together. Susan admits that a leaky pouch might startle her, but she doesn't see it as a catastrophe. It certainly wouldn't change her love for Jim. After all, they've been through a lot together, including a long siege of illness. Now it's time to delight in his returning health. They've decided that for now they'll just enjoy each other, talking, hugging, touching for the pure pleasure of it without a further goal in mind. Spontaneously, Jim hugs Susan and. . .

Actually, the first experience with lovemaking after surgery can be great, disappointing, or anything in between. Like one's first experience with sex, it may have more of nerves than of love in it. Yet, if they relax a bit, both partners can enjoy a warm, pleasurable, and rewarding intimacy. Sex, after all, is not performance but sharing.

Probably the most basic factor in sexual intimacy is liking oneself. That feeling of being a worthwhile person, with or without an ostomy, becomes contagious. If we feel good about ourselves, others feel good about us too. If we accept an ostomy, others accept it too. Even in ideal circumstances, it takes time: to become comfortable with a new ostomy, to forget it most of the time, to return to being a person who just happens to have an ostomy, rather than an ostomy with a person attached. Most of us have some doubts about ourselves, even before ostomy surgery. When these doubts are severe enough to interfere with our lives, it's time for professional help.

Jennifer, for instance, was a very attractive single woman, who had had her ileostomy for three years. Her friends were baffled: They introduced pretty, bright, nice Jennifer to young men, but nothing happened. As she was able to laugh about it later, after some therapy, there was a simple explanation. So terrified was she that a date would find out about her ostomy that she froze if he took her hand. If a man put his arm around her, she leaped up with a fragile excuse. She maneuvered her date to the side away from her ostomy. She constantly covered her pouch with her right arm. So frightened was she that a man would find out about her ostomy that she didn't give him a chance to find out about any part of her.

After a few sessions of therapy, Jennifer discovered that she'd used the ostomy as a scapegoat for all the doubts she'd had about herself before surgery. As she became happier about herself, she no longer had to spend all her energy protecting her ostomy—and herself—from discovery. Secure in herself, she was free to learn about other people. (Her last Christmas card mentioned that she and Eric had just celebrated their fifth anniversary; her other big news was the birth of Steven in October.)

Communication is the next critical factor in any sexual meeting. This raises the question: When do I tell him (or her) about my ostomy? "When discovery is imminent"— though a popular answer—may not be the best.

When ostomy surgery happens during a serious ongoing relationship, the partner will probably know all about it from the beginning. But what about a new romance?

As a general rule, the person with an ostomy should tell, at the latest, when it seems possible that intimacy is likely to occur. Before marriage, certainly. Some people feel so much more at ease with their dates *after* they tell them that they make a practice of explaining the ostomy quite early in the friendship.

A simple explanation is sufficient. Basically, the person who has an ileostomy, for instance, could say something like this: "I trust you enough to tell you this. I was very sick for a long time. Finally, to save my life, I had serious surgery. I'm perfectly healthy now. But the surgeons made a change in my plumbing—they removed my colon and rectum—and now I go to the bathroom differently. I wear a special pouch, so now I can finally do all the things I want to do." If questions follow, the person answers them, clearly, simply, honestly and confidently.

Marlene Vine met her husband in college. "After we had been going together for some time I realized it was time I told him about my ileostomy. I thought, 'Gee, I don't know how he's going to react.' I was so nervous—I had built up such a huge thing in my mind. When I was ready to tell him, he turned to me and said: 'Yes, I know.' That was the last thing I expected to hear!"

At the time, Marlene had worn a rather clumsy pouch, which her boyfriend had felt while embracing her. Bewildered, he had checked with a doctor and then with the library, so that he knew all about the operation before Marlene got around to telling him.

One woman resolved the "how to tell" dilemma by informing her boyfriend, "I can't go out with you Sunday afternoon. I have a meeting to attend. Would you like to come with me?"—then taking him to the local UOA meeting!

Most partners who are otherwise right for each other come to accept the ostomy, but it may take time. Mary Ryan admits she was husband-hunting when she met a "very distinguished gentleman." The friendship thrived, until one evening he told her he had a colostomy: "As I remember, I was very calm and polite, my only feelings at the moment being for him and what an unfortunate situation this must be." She agonized for two days, filled with foreboding and doubts, then visited a nurse's office down the hall from her own office.

"The nurse very briskly and efficiently described a colostomy, even drawing me a picture. She wanted to know my reasons in detail and finished our session with these words of wisdom, 'If this bothers you about an otherwise eligible and fine person, you deserve not even the shadow of a thought from him again.' "

The nurse's insult cleared the air and Mary was able to talk frankly with her man friend instead of working so hard to be consciously kind.

"His insistence that we analyze how I felt about it became masterfully appealing. His honesty, his compassion for me in adjusting to this unknown, and his own basic good sense that a wife-to-be should thoroughly understand, lighted our way. I passed the test with this well-planned tutelage. And, I am proud and happy to say I have the finest, most loving husband in the world."

Although Mary's exploration took time, the resulting understanding became another bond between them.

Ostomy surgery, particularly after long illness, may bring to the surface turbulent, mixed feelings in the partner. Ben Frankel, trying to keep his law practice, two small children and multiple bills in order during his wife's long hospitalization, tells of the painful and ambivalent feelings he faced: "I think underlying it all was the tremendous feeling that I had of anger and resentment that Judy was doing this to me and our family. At the time those feelings started to come up I couldn't really express them, because I knew it was not appropriate for me to feel that way—those were wrong, bad feelings. I had to kind of put them down because you are not allowed to feel angry at your wife because she's sick. I felt angry about the anger, but felt angry anyway! The passage of time helped overcome the feelings of this sort, along with expressing the feelings to yourself first and to other members of your family."

It took a huge argument and a brief separation to clear the air for the Frankels. Until partners can accept these feelings in themselves, communicate them, and begin working together to resolve them, their sex life may suffer. Recognizing that such feelings are normal and common makes them easier to face.

Some partners take longer than Mary and Ben did to accept an ostomy, some less time, and there are a few who never accept it. Either the person with the ostomy or the partner may curtail or even end a sexual relationship, giving the ostomy as the reason; sometimes it's an excuse, a way to camouflage bigger problems. If things don't improve after a reasonable length of time and more information, both partners need to decide if what they share is worth saving. Counseling may help sort out tangled feelings if both want to continue together.

When, as does happen occasionally, a partner does reject a person with an ostomy, the experience can be devastating. As hard as it is to keep the situation in perspective at the time, it's essential for the person to remember that he or she is still desirable, still basically the same person as before surgery—and that it is the partner's loss.

Usually though, perhaps after a period of shock and grieving by both partners, a rewarding intimacy can survive—and grow—after ostomy surgery. It's unlikely that such surgery would glue a poor relationship together. But it's even more doubtful that such a change in one's personal plumbing could weaken a sturdy relationship. Many couples have reported a new closeness. Partners find out how much they do mean to each other and rejoice in discovering how much they can grow.

A few suggestions about down-to-earth matters may be useful.

Baths and showers are good not only for the stoma area but for sex appeal. Cleanliness is sexy. Even when spontaneity overrides everything else, there's usually time to check that the appliance is clean, empty, and firmly adhered. Most people who wear pouches at other times wear them during lovemaking also. A colostomy plug is an option for some people with sigmoid colostomies.

A slight amount of camouflage may be welcome. Pouch covers can be purchased or easily stitched at home from a small scrap of fabric. Some people prefer to tuck the appliance under a belt or cummerbund. A number of women, inspired by sexy lingerie catalogs, purchase pretty opaque panties and split the middle of the crotch to about five inches (12 cm) below the waistline, front and back. Cut edges are hemmed and sometimes trimmed with lace or other decoration. (The *Ostomy Quarterly* often carries advertisements for attractive lingerie.)

It helps to know, and to assure one's partner, that the stoma won't get hurt during sexplay (although it is not recommended as a receptive organ in intercourse because of the high risk of injury). It may bleed a few drops if it gets bumped because there are many blood vessels near the surface, but that can be safely ignored. Sometimes a partner may wish to see the stoma, sometimes not. A good time is under the shower, or in the bathtub.

Depending on stoma location and pouch, some lovemaking positions may be more comfortable than others. That's where speaking up is important.

Keeping one's sense of humor handy smoothes the way if the unexpected happens. If an appliance slips or a stoma becomes musical at an inappropriate moment, so what? People who don't have ostomies also pass gas or belch at inappropriate times. A shared laugh, and the world continues to spin.

Something like 50% of all married couples report sex difficulties of one kind or another, and people with ostomies are not exempt. Many problems can be solved with tenderness, patience, clear talk, and a little more information. Sex counselors can provide the facts; so can reputable sexual manuals. Some doctors are comfortable and knowledgeable about sexual matters; some, unfortunately, are not. ET nurses, thanks to experience with the problems of many couples, can give information and encouragement. They can help make clear, for instance, that the person with a new ostomy may be apathetic about sex for a time after surgery, until the stoma and the new body image are accepted. While the partner needs to be sensitive to this, some initiative may help in conveying the message that this new image is OK.

Although much of sex may be mental, there still can be physical problems after ostomy surgery. A number of women who have had the rectum removed report painful intercourse for weeks or months after surgery; in most cases, there is a remarkable and satisfying improvement, although it may take time for muscles, nerves, and blood vessels disturbed during surgery to get back to normal. This is a temporary problem; the best remedies are patience, time, gentleness, enough stimulation, and letting one's partner know what feels good.

In the rare case where a woman undergoes extensive surgery of the pelvis with removal of vagina and clitoris as well as of uterus, bowel and bladder, she faces obvious problems. Even in this case, if it's important enough to the individual, plastic surgery may help with physical reconstruction although sensation in the area will be changed or gone.

For men, the situation is more complicated. There are four parts to a man's sexual response: erection, ejaculation, orgasm and fertility. No ostomy surgery rules out the possibility of orgasm. Some kinds of surgery, however, may interfere with erection, ejaculation or fertility.

Since the psychological and the physical intertwine in the process of erection, it may take a urologist to decide whether a particular problem results from anxiety or from surgical damage. Most people with ileostomies find that such problems are temporary. The more radical surgery for cancer causes more damage; some people who undergo ostomy surgery for cancer report a permanent inability to have an erection, although many others have no problems.

Even when the condition is temporary, a person may wait months or even years as nerve damage heals before regaining the ability to have an erection. Ed Ward, a past president of UOA who has a colostomy, waited 2 1/2 years. His wife, Anne, hadn't met him then but (as she tells it) ". . .he tells me that regeneration came about gradually. By the time we were married, almost five years following his surgery, he was well within the realm of normal for which we are both grateful. Had he remained impotent, I really don't think it would have made a difference. We love each other dearly and although physical love is important, it is not the only deciding factor in a good marriage. There are many ways to express physical love or to fulfill emotional needs. A tender word, a squeeze of the hand, or a glance across a crowded room are all expressions of love."

A urologist is the one to advise the man about problems with erection. He's also the one who has information about penile implants, one of the newer surgical solutions to physiological problems with erection. So many men with other medical conditions (diabetes, for instance) cannot achieve an erection that implant surgery is a developing field. Some men have found this mechanical assistance quite satisfactory. Slender rods or inflatable cylinders are inserted on both sides of the penis; new techniques are appearing all the time. Insurance may or may not cover the operation.

Another possible solution is vacuum therapy. Before intercourse, the man places his non-erect penis into a plastic cylinder attached to a small pump which creates a vacuum, pulling additional blood into the penis to enlarge it. After the penis becomes erect, a band temporarily placed around the base of the penis keeps the additional blood in place during intercourse. After intercourse, the band is removed and the penis returns to its normal non-erect size.

Another treatment, the Pharmacological Erection Program (PEP) has the man use small syringes and needles (the same kind a diabetic uses) to inject the penis before intercourse. One medicine opens up the arteries into the penis so that more blood flows in, while a second clamps down the veins that drain the penis so that the blood stays in the penis for an hour or two.

A few medical centers are experimenting with operations which bring a small artery into the penis to increase the blood supply for erection. These are called revascularization surgeries.

The grapevine sometimes reports on home remedies for sexual problems—such as a rubber band at the base of the penis for those who can achieve but not maintain an erection. Such self-help can cause serious problems if done incorrectly; a urologist or other knowledgeable health professional can show the safe way to do it.

Probably most people in the world could multiply their pleasure by broadening their sexual horizons—and that includes anyone with erection difficulty. The genitals are not the only erogenous zone: The whole body is an immense sensual and sexual network which few of us ever explore fully. All the body can respond to caresses, tenderness and passion. Skin has been called the largest sex organ in the body—and with good reason. Other varieties of sexual experience can bring deep pleasure. A good sex manual can provide details.

Many men who have had ostomy surgery because of cancer, find that they no longer ejaculate, even if they have erections and orgasms. The body handles this change easily, but it may take time for the mind and emotions to adjust.

If a man hopes to father a child after ostomy surgery for cancer, he may want to check with a urologist before surgery about storing his sperm for later artificial insemination. However, after surgery, couples who wish to avoid pregnancy still need a reliable contraceptive, unless testing confirms a zero sperm count.

Premenopausal women can definitely get pregnant after ostomy surgery—and frequently do, bearing healthy babies. The woman who does not want to get pregnant needs to check that her birth control pill is not passing whole into the pouch. If it is, it's time for another method of contraception.

Ostomy surgery does not change sexual realities. All men and women, with or without ostomies, need to protect themselves from the dangers of sexually-transmitted diseases, including AIDS.

Some groups of people have particular concerns after ostomy surgery. Single men and women, for instance, can attend their own events at annual United Ostomy Association conferences, meet other singles, and compare experiences and strategies. The Gay and Lesbian Concerns Committee of UOA provides seminars, brochures, and other help and mutual support for homosexuals and bisexuals who have ostomies. Information about these special interest groups is available from UOA.

In spite of *Playboy* stereotypes, it is wise for everyone—with or without an ostomy—to think of love and sex in the broadest terms, and to be willing to try alternative ways of achieving satisfaction. If it feels good for the two people involved, it is good. There are no standards of comparison. Life is ours to live and enjoy. Sex, always expressed in one way or another, is part of that enjoyment.

"The important thing," adds Dr. Lawrence P. Davis, "is not to make your appliance a chastity belt."

CHAPTER 19 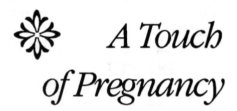 *A Touch of Pregnancy*

> *To heir is human.*
> Dolores E. McGuire

"But can I have a baby?"

The young woman queries her doctor, buttonholes the nurse, corners the ET nurse or the ostomy visitor: "Can I have a baby despite my ostomy?"

The answer in almost all cases is a thundering *yes!* Although women with ostomies may choose to skip peanuts or chop suey, there is usually no reason to avoid pregnancy if they want a baby. Women with ostomies are getting pregnant and delivering healthy babies all the time. First babies. Twins. Several babies.

Corrine Barnes, from the Maryland area, claims that when she volunteered as an ostomy visitor, talking with young women before or soon after ostomy surgery, she heard the question often—and gave the standard answer, that surgery itself does not prevent pregnancy. She goes on to say: "While this is true, it does leave something to be desired as an answer to a very serious question. Now I have a more positive response, and that is that seven years following my ileostomy, I can confirm that pregnancy is very definitely possible. Our first child, Teresa, was born at Holy Cross. . . .[Then] Teresa's brother Timothy was born."

"Apprehension during pregnancy is certainly not uncommon," writes Janice Hoppes, of Manhattan, Montana, "but don't let an ostomy be your big worry. This, my first pregnancy, proved to be a time of many unfounded fears. With good prenatal care your pregnancy will be as normal as any woman's."

In fact, knowing that women with ostomies can have safe, comfortable, happy pregnancies and deliveries is half the battle. Dr. Albert S. Lyons helped organize one of the first mutual aid groups for people with ostomies in New York in 1951. He recalls: "When our first ileostomate had a normal delivery, the women in our fledgling ostomy group went flip-flop. Their bellies began expanding. . . ."

Paul Zeit, MD, draws on years of experience as an obstetrician in a large referral clinic when he reassures doctors and prospective parents: ". . .One learns three very important facts that are not generally understood by most obstetricians, by many surgeons, and by most women who have ostomies of one sort or another. The first fact is that patients with stomas present no different obstetrical problems than patients without stomas. Second, the pregnancy does not create any new surgical problems and it does not alter bowel function in ostomates any more than it does in women with an intact gastrointestinal tract. Third, there are amazingly few mechanical problems with appliances that are brought about by pregnancy."

Doctors tend to advise a wait of a year or two after surgery before conception. Some women, of course, become pregnant before then and generally have uneventful pregnancies, but the body appreciates a chance to heal fully from surgery, to toughen abdominal muscles which may be lazy, and to rebuild nutritional reserves that may have been depleted by bowel disease before surgery. Too, the mother-to-be needs a chance to get accustomed to her stoma before taking on a new baby—plus time to adjust to a new body image before changing it again with pregnancy.

Once a man and woman decide they want a child and are reasonably well-prepared for parenthood, a check with the doctor comes next. A phone conversation or visit may be enough to answer questions, to quiet fears. The prospective parents, for instance, learn that even drastic bowel surgery, like removal of one-third to one-half of the small bowel, shouldn't jeopardize the baby's food supply before birth; most food absorption takes place in the first half of the small intestine.

There are a few special cases, of course. A man or woman with ostomy surgery for familial polyps needs to know that any children are at risk for polyposis and may require bowel surgery during young adulthood. Women with urinary ostomies must take special precautions against urinary tract infection during pregnancy. Women with ostomies for cancer, especially those who have undergone radiation and/or chemotherapy, need counseling from their doctors.

Some women have difficulty becoming pregnant or carrying a baby to term, but neither inflammatory bowel disease nor ostomy surgery is ordinarily a cause. Fertility clinics and/or obstetricians who specialize in high risk pregnancies are possible resources.

Finding the right doctor for pregnancy and delivery— before conception, if possible—takes thought. This applies to every woman, with or without an ostomy. Some women already have a doctor in whom they have confidence. Others may follow the recommendation of a friend (possibly of a friend with an ostomy who has had a baby since surgery), or of their internist or surgeon, or of a teaching hospital in the area. Many doctors have never been present when a woman with an ostomy delivers her child—but this doesn't seem to matter much. As Mary Bir, from Great Lakes, Illinois, warns: "Don't be surprised if your doctor says something like mine did, 'Oh! We don't get too many of your kind.'"

More important than experience with ostomies are the doctor's skill, sensitivity and supportiveness. The doctor who's initially a greenhorn about ostomies can do an expert job, with a little help, perhaps, from the woman's internist or surgeon and from the literature. And many of the general questions which bubble forth from most prospective parents—what about natural childbirth? breastfeeding? fees?—are far more important than the ostomy-related queries.

The woman with an ostomy who becomes pregnant actually enjoys some advantages over those who won't have ostomies. Writes Mary Bir: "I had a child before and after my surgery. Personally I enjoyed the latter pregnancy much more than my first. One of the many things I did not have to worry about was hemorrhoids and constipation." In fact, if a large piece of intestine has been removed, there's more room for the growing fetus. Women with ostomies are not immune, however, from the common experiences of pregnancy, like morning sickness, fatigue alternating with surges of energy, mood swings. And they need to remember the rules which apply to any pregnancy: nutritious diet, regular check-ups, reasonable weight gain.

"There is no reason," states Dr. Zeit, "why she can't carry a pregnancy to term without any more restrictions on her activities than any other woman. . . ."

Ann Wolf confirms Zeit's statement: "My pregnancy was quite uneventful. I continued to work until four weeks before my due date. Then I was so bored at home that I began a new job and even worked the day before the baby was born. We also began packing our belongings because three weeks before my due date we sold our home and had thirty days to move out! We didn't even have a place to move to. So all at once we were packing, looking for a house, and having a baby. Finally we found a house and moved when the baby was only two weeks old." (What does she call an *eventful* pregnancy?)

Some specifics: Many pregnant women with ostomies find themselves needing more fluids than before. They may notice a change in the consistency of stool, which may become either more liquid or thicker. On some rare occasions, near the end of pregnancy, the uterus will press enough on the intestine to cause a mechanical obstruction; a change of position or, if necessary, a liquid or soft diet for a time solves that problem.

To help prevent or lessen stretch marks, pregnant women can rub a non-oily moisturizer around the incision and all over the belly during that nine months stretch (if moisturizer is used right around the stoma, it needs to be a kind that doesn't interfere with pouch adhesion.) The doctor may recommend an ointment or lotion for the perineal wound, if any. (Some surgeons, anticipating childbirth, leave the rectum intact during the childbearing years so there is no perineal wound; many obstetricians claim that the perineal scar becomes so elastic during pregnancy that it causes no problems during childbirth.)

Pregnant women with ostomies report remarkably little change in the stoma. Generally it becomes elongated, somewhat oval-shaped, and may require a different sized faceplate opening or a reshaped skin barrier. The stoma may increase slightly in diameter temporarily, may protrude a bit more, and, as the blood supply increases to an already well-supplied area, it may bleed slightly. A bigger problem is centering the pouch as baby and belly grow. Some women suggest a full length mirror—or a mate's help—and perhaps some paper centering guides for that maneuver. Skin tends to get oilier as pregnancy progresses and some women change pouches more often if adhesion is a problem. Babies also kick around the stoma on occasion; this can cause a little soreness but no real harm.

Women with continent ileostomies have had normal pregnancies and deliveries, without difficulty. Irwin Gelernt, MD, finds that "the only thing that happens is that the reservoir needs to be emptied more often as the enlarging womb compresses the reservoir. The angle of intubation also changes slightly, but there is no real difficulty with this new angle."

When it's time to go to the hospital, it's wise to bring and display prominently a card with basic information on it: the kind of ostomy, and do's and don'ts—especially no enemas, no rectal temperatures (for the women who has had her rectum and anus removed). Janice Hoppes expressed her thanks to her thoughtful obstetrician who alerted the small hospital where she planned to deliver her baby so they could brush up on their ileostomy care before she arrived. But not all hospital staffs are so prepared, and a woman may need to remind a staff member of basic information about ostomies.

How about delivery? Is a Caesarean section necessary? Dr. Zeit says firmly: "There is no reason for a higher Caesarean section rate in these women than in any other group of women."

Many women, with or without ostomies, wonder if the perineal region will tear during a vaginal delivery. Major problems are rare. Labor and delivery don't harm the stoma or the abdominal incision either.

Some women wear their reusable pouch through labor and delivery while others prefer disposables, bypassing the washing and hanging routine during those hectic early days of motherhood. In those first days there may be a problem maintaining a good seal, since the abdominal contour changes drastically and the skin tends to be flabby for a while. If leakage occurs, the doctor or ET nurse can suggest remedies.

Janice Hoppes found that she could handle her ostomy care herself after delivery, and was much less embarrassed than she expected to be by such things as her appliance showing while she dressed after showering: "Remember, on an obstetrical floor the only really noticeable objects are the babies in the nursery!

". . .I continued to change my appliance every two days for approximately two weeks following delivery due to my shrinking abdomen to prevent any excoriation. My stoma remains elongated, but the base has returned to its original size."

Concludes Janice: "As a side note on labor and delivery, all new mothers spend time visiting. It was the general consensus that I had probably had the least complicated labor and delivery of any of us. So you can see that an ostomy does not prove to be a barrier during the nine months of pregnancy, nor during the labor and delivery."

CHAPTER 20 ✿ *Children with Ostomies*

Natalie Berenstein of Bexley, Ohio, was six years old when she offered some advice to other children with ostomies: "This is what I would tell another girl or boy about to have an ostomy: Don't be scared about it. Don't get upset. You'll do fine, and you can do anything that you want to do with it!"

Natalie said it well. Many doctors, ET nurses and parents of children with stomas would echo her:

CHILDREN WHO NEED OSTOMIES—AND GET THEM—ARE THE LUCKY ONES AND DO WONDERFULLY WELL!

Babies just a few hours old undergo ostomy surgery—and thrive. Preschoolers, given a chance, learn to manage appliances almost as efficiently as their elders—although they may occasionally attach a pouch upside down!

Natalie's surgery was done because of spinal damage present at birth; at the time she advised other children with ostomies, she was swimming, riding her bike, playing on the bars of the playgym and working out on a trampoline.

Other children may be born with defects in bladder, bowel or anus that require either a permanent or a temporary ostomy. Disease (ulcerative colitis, for instance) or injury may make surgery necessary. If a child suffers repeated kidney infections because of a defect in the urinary tract, an ostomy may be done to protect the endangered kidneys from further damage. And, as a last resort in cases of incontinence, an ostomy may free a child from endless diapers and plastic pants.

For parents, the news their young child will have an ostomy usually comes as a shattering blow. Shannon Vyff, of Wichita, Kansas, was born without certain important nerves of the descending colon. After trying different treatments, Shannon's pediatric surgeon suggested exploratory surgery to confirm the diagnosis; if the nerves were abnormal, he planned to give Shannon a temporary colostomy. Shannon's mother Janice relives that devastating time: "As the time during the operation dragged on my spirits fell. It took so long, I just knew she had undergone colostomy surgery. I was right. She received her first colostomy, in the descending colon, at four months and one week of age.

"I was so upset. I couldn't stand the idea of my beautiful little daughter being so 'disfigured' in this manner. If my husband had not been there to give me his help and support, I don't know what I might have done. I remained quite bitter about the surgery for a few days.

"Then, at Dr. Mirza's request, a wonderful lady, Rose Randall [who had an ostomy], came to visit us at the hospital. . . . I decided that if Rose could be so great, an ostomy on Shannon might not be so awful after all.

"And it wasn't! I learned to like Shannon's colostomy, because it made her so comfortable. She immediately started sleeping through the night. Her personality completely changed, and she became an extremely happy baby."

For a time, many urinary diversions were done so a child could be dry. The pendulum has swung to other solutions, when possible: medicines, bladder massage techniques, intermittent-catheterization (inserting a tube into the bladder several times a day to drain urine). But sometimes an ostomy is the only answer.

Mrs. Larry Case, of Morgan City, Louisiana, reflects on the pain and indecision of the parent forced to make the decision about elective ostomy surgery in a child. Her son Rob had been plagued with bladder and kidney problems since he was five. When the surgery was scheduled, she panicked—as numerous parents do, especially those who have never met and talked with anyone with an ostomy— and canceled the operation. "At my request his doctor came and my son made the decision that he wanted to be dry. He felt that he would be more like other children that way. I still didn't reschedule the surgery and I had the most terrible week of my life. I suffered for my son's life ahead; the problems he would encounter. Whenever he slept, I cried like it was the end of the world."

Happily, mother and son met a little girl in the x-ray waiting room and discovered that her ostomy pouch didn't show under her dress. But Mrs. Case agonized: "Anyway, I resigned myself to my son's terrible fate. I was assured that in a relatively short time he would be able to care for himself. I didn't have any confidence in this either. I was completely negative. I had no one or nowhere to turn.

"The moral of this story is that all our fears were proved wrong by the one who never had fear. This tiny little boy, who had always been small because he was always so sick, never gave anyone the opportunity to consider him handicapped. He has always been an honor student even with the amount of school he's missed. He is a very good golfer, plays tennis, swims, plays shortstop in Little League and is an outstanding Biddy Basketball player."

Once the go-ahead comes from doctor and parents for ostomy surgery, what then? For the infant in diapers, parents, or the person who usually cares for the child, step in to learn about care. Since the child is already in diapers, there may be no big change in the care—except that the diaper may be a little higher! (The child with an ostomy which produces a liquid stool will need a small pouch to protect the skin from enzymes.)

Preschoolers and young school-age children begin to learn how to care for themselves. Jean Alvers, ET, uses a puppet theater to show children what will be happening to them. Play therapy, in which children practice putting pouches on dolls and coping with common problems, helps them vent their own feelings, and increases security in this new situation. *Chris has an Ostomy*, a booklet available from UOA, helps children understand. Meeting another child with an ostomy can be invaluable for an older child; if that's not possible, talking to an adult with an ostomy can reassure both child and parents.

Children accept glasses or braces. Just as naturally do they seem to accept ostomies.

Not only parents but older children, grandparents, and babysitters also can learn the basics of caring for the young child's ostomy. This "thing," which seemed at first so horrendous, gradually becomes commonplace and no longer frightening. "Is that all there is to it?" becomes the new question.

Skin care and pouch use require a little special attention with children. Stoma size changes as the child grows and pouches need to be checked for fit frequently. Children may need a few gentle reminders not to skimp on skin care, if they are taking charge of their own ostomies. Basically, as for anyone with an ostomy, the appliance-wearing child needs intact skin, a pouch which fits, and a good seal to prevent leakage and promote security. Small pouches, made especially for young children, are available commercially. (For bathtime or other splashing, adding waterproof tape around the appliance can cut down on pouch changes.)

Many ostomies for young children are temporary, often to bypass the bowel or part of the urinary tract until the child is large enough for corrective surgery (see *Chapter 14—Temporary Ostomies.*) The expert help of an ET nurse can untangle the problems of caring for these ostomies. When the temporary ostomy isn't needed any more, the reconnection surgery is called *undiversion*, because the intestine or urinary tract is no longer diverted.

When can a child start caring for an ostomy? In general, children can start assuming responsibility at the toilet training age; if they have ostomy surgery after two or three, they can begin immediately. Emptying the pouch comes first. Then, as the child becomes more mature and dexterous, he or she learns about changing pouches, maintaining the skin, and checking for any problems. Complete independence is the goal. The very young who require assistance receive it, of course, but soon learn to distinguish between a helping hand and having all the care done for them.

As children grow, they strive for adulthood. Dressing themselves, learning to cross the street, and going to school are all steps on this path to gradual independence. So is caring for an ostomy. The parent who continues to care for a child's ostomy past a reasonable age because it's "faster" or "easier" or "better" that way, gives the child the message that he or she "can't do it right." Tying a shoelace may be a challenge when one is five—and so is changing a pouch—but well worth doing.

Parents can help by simplifying procedures and gathering equipment in a place the child can reach. Beyond that, their greatest contribution is in teaching patiently and lovingly—and then stepping back so the child can assume responsibility and the pride that comes with it.

Naomi Remen, MD, who has an ileostomy herself and is a pediatrician at Stanford University, reminds parents of their crucial role in helping the child with the ostomy: "It is important that the family think of the child as a well child. This is difficult, as often the child has been ill for many months or even years. Now, after his surgery, he is well, and both he and his family must begin to think of him as a competent and total human being. The ostomy and its care should never be used as an excuse for special treatment or privilege. The child should be thought of as a child with, say, glasses or dental braces. These appliances need to be considered in playing sports or traveling, but the consideration should be routine and matter-of-fact."

In some cases, of course, the child has underlying disease, perhaps a spinal defect. But after surgery, the child is better. He or she can start meeting the world in ways not possible before the ostomy.

Dr. Remen acknowledges that parents of children with ostomies may have a hard time making their own adjustments: "They may feel a loss of self-esteem as the parents of a 'defective' child and see the ostomy as a 'flaw' in an otherwise 'perfect' son or daughter. They may feel guilt over what they think is a painful problem they have genetically transmitted to a small child. They may feel resentment towards the child for the worry he has caused and the disruption of family life his illness has represented. They may also resent the financial burden that the illness has imposed on them.

". . .Such feelings are common and every attempt must be made to work them through and not communicate them to the child. We learn self-love and self-esteem from our parents. Children are maimed by non-accepting parents and not by a surgical procedure which opens for them the opportunity of a healthy and full life."

The doctor, ET nurses, other health personnel, and religious counselors or psychotherapists—any may be helpful for parents trying to sort out such feelings.

Dr. Remen suggests open discussion of the ostomy among family and friends of all ages. Concealing the fact may make the child feel ashamed or even maimed. Stories about themselves—how they were sick, how Mommy and Daddy felt, how the doctors helped make them well with the surgery—together with simple, clear explanations of what an ostomy is, are very popular with the younger set.

If the child feels good about himself, a reflection at this young age of the parents' good feelings about the child, he or she is in fine shape to handle any minor storms that arise. Schoolmates and young friends generally accept the situation—often with a little envy! As Rob Case's mother reports: "Other parents have chosen to handle this another way, but being from a small town there was no way for Rob's condition to be a secret. It has worked out beautifully for Rob. All of his friends know, but I don't think they give it a second thought. The mother of one of his classmates told me that her child came home well pleased because 'Rob had a new bag and it sure was pretty.' My six-year-old son says he'd like one also."

It makes sense to inform the school-age child's teacher and school nurse about the ostomy. An extra pouch set-up can be left at school in case of a leak.

Meeting other children with ostomies, if possible, at ostomy association meetings or through the doctor, ET nurse, or other health personnel (who may know other children with similar surgery), helps immensely, especially for any child who encounters a problem.

The UOA headquarters office is the place to call about support networks and groups for parents of children with ostomies or incontinence and for the children themselves. (United Ostomy Association, Inc., 36 Executive Park, Suite 120, Irvine, California, 92714-6744, Telephone: 1-800-826-0826.) Some are geared toward specific groups (parents of children with bowel ostomies or problems, for instance) while others are more general. If there is no group nearby, support can be by phone or letter (or it may be possible to start a group.)

These are a way for parents and children to learn they are not alone, not the only ones coping with these peculiar changes in personal plumbing. Networks and groups can be a source of moral support, practical hints on what has worked for other people, and information on what's new in treatment and equipment. How do I get the skin dry enough for the pouch to stick when urine keeps dribbling out all the time? What are the latest surgical techniques for my child who was born with no anal opening for stool? What do I say to my son who wants to sit on the potty chair like his friends—but has a urostomy and a colostomy? Joining together can also help bring about change in the outside world, whether it's child-sized pouches, new insurance legislation, or a community which knows more about these children.

Stacy, a very young lady from Evansville, Indiana, sports two ostomies: an ileostomy and a urostomy. Stacy's mother reports: "Being a very inquisitive child, Stacy has naturally started asking a few questions about her ostomies. We just answer her honestly and simply; she accepts that and is satisfied—just as we, our family and friends have accepted her ostomies, and in fact, count them as blessings. We know that because of her ostomies she is now leading a completely normal and VERY active life."

CHAPTER 21 ❄ *A Word to the Teenagers*

Having a colostomy doesn't stop a person from living and enjoying life. I'm not afraid to tell anyone about my ostomy, nor should it be made taboo. I can now eat anything I want. I love salads, fruits, pizzas, etc. I can enjoy every thing. I have a girl friend, in fact more than one.

Mark Singer

Mark Singer, of Metro Maryland Youth Ostomy Association, didn't always accept his ostomy so happily. When doctors told him they planned a colostomy for his Crohn's disease, Mark balked: "I thought it was the worst thing that could happen to anyone. When I heard the word and the way it was put to me I wanted to die."

Jim Clark went a little further. He accepted surgery (he thought) and then tried to check out of the hospital the night before his operation was scheduled: "I was so scared. . . . So they notified security and security picked me up at the gate. I was kind of obvious, because I was the only one wearing a nightgown!" Even after he was returned to his room, Jim barricaded the door.

What made the difference for both Mark and Jim was meeting a person who had an ostomy. Mark's mother called the local ostomy chapter; an ostomy visitor came to see Mark every day before surgery and every day afterwards. For Jim, it was a person whom the hospital contacted after Jim's attempted escape. He showed up right before Jim's surgery: "I always thought that ostomates were green people who were really wild, but he was a normal-looking person and he came to see me at four o'clock in the morning to wish me good luck. That's all I needed. . . ."

Many young people have ostomies. Some have had them since they were babies. Some choose an ostomy as they grow up after struggling for years with constant wetness and diapers for a birth defect or other urinary tract problem that couldn't be corrected any other way. A few teenagers have ostomies after an accident in which their bowel or urinary tract is injured. But most young people who undergo ostomy surgery have ulcerative colitis or Crohn's disease.

When you've been sick for a long time with a bowel disease, you may be so anxious to get rid of the pain and misery that you really don't care much how it happens. But an *ostomy?* Having to wear a "bag" everywhere? That sounds even worse than the disease. Especially when you're weak and sick, that may seem like the last straw.

That's how it seemed to Naomi Remen. She had an ileostomy at 17 for ulcerative colitis, although she couldn't stand even the thought of an ostomy and decided not to learn how to put on a pouch. Secretly, she plotted to kill herself upon leaving the hospital. But after she went home, she received a phone call from a woman who was a member of the local ostomy association. Naomi refused to see her, but the persistent woman said she would come anyway. One look at a beautiful woman in a tight skirt—and Naomi decided life might be worth living after all. (She eventually became a pediatrician, and frequently writes articles about ostomies and young people.)

There *are* special problems for teenagers. You're trying to find out just who you are. You want to be yourself, an individual, but not too different from everyone else. It's not easy to think of yourself as a normal, healthy person when you're sick all the time. An ostomy can make you a healthy person again, but it's hard, at first, to keep from feeling really different from everyone else. When you first have an ostomy, it's difficult to convince yourself that other people aren't aware of it unless you tell them. But once you've learned the basics of caring for an ostomy, other people don't need to know. An ostomy is much easier to hide than acne or a pudgy middle.

One of the big hassles for a lot of young people is becoming independent. Accepting the authority of doctors and parents to make decisions about *you* (for instance that you need an ostomy) can raise the rebel in any teenager. When you've been sick a long time, you may find it hard after ostomy surgery to get parents to accept the fact that you're healthy now and can start having more say in your life. On the other hand, when you've been used to some special attention and pleasant coddling, you may not feel like giving it up. Sometimes, people (of any age) who live with a chronic problem like inflammatory bowel disease become true con artists at getting other people to meet their needs and wishes; it takes effort and desire to learn healthier and more fun ways of living with others.

Some days all teenagers wish they could be young children again, with parents caring for their every need. Other days they'd like to be completely grown up and on their own with no one telling them what to do. This emotional teeter-tottering is just part of growing up, although that doesn't make it any easier to accept.

Often it's hard to understand how parents feel,

especially when you have your hands full already coping with your own problems—one of which is probably parents! Some parents feel guilty because you've been sick; they may wonder if they might have prevented it by doing something differently. Since a lot of parents are reluctant to see their children grow up and away from them, they may want to baby you, either during illness or after an ostomy. Some parents have difficulty accepting any disease or problem in their "perfect" children. Other parents may harbor resentments about the emotional and financial drains the illness has made on them; these are normal feelings, no matter how much parents love a child but, since most parents would feel guilty about expressing them directly, the resentment crops up in strange places where it can really hurt.

Sometimes it's *really* hard to decipher the meaning behind what a parent says. One participant at a Youth Rap Session at a UOA Conference faced such a parent problem: "I went out on a date with a young man and when I came back my father said: 'Did you have a good time?' And I said: 'Yes, blah, blah, blah—this is where we went, this is what we did.' My father said: 'Too bad he can't afford the medical bills, isn't it.'

"Right after your surgery, you have this new little thing there on your side, and you are wondering how people are going to accept you; what you are going to do. You go out on a date and you come back and your dad says that, it's like putting you back about six months."

As devastating as the father's comment was—and many a parent has made some similar statement to a teenager, with or without an ostomy—one of the subtler messages behind the words actually may be something like this: "I, your father, *can* pay your medical bills. I may not be as young and handsome as this kid, but I'm still your dad and I'll take care of you. . . ." Growing up means becoming independent of parents and that rarely happens smoothly.

There are bumps and curves along the way, for all teenagers, all parents.

Especially after a long illness, you may feel like Rip Van Winkle re-entering the world. Even if you participated in school and activities during the illness before an ostomy, so much of your energy was tied up with being sick, that it was kind of a half-hearted participation. Young people are not known for their patience, and this period of catching up—with school, with social life, with thinking about a career—isn't easy. One good friend can help a lot, as can a school counselor or a favorite teacher. There are a lot of people willing to help.

Just about every teenager experiences rejection by someone, at some time, for some reason. A few people may not accept you because of the ostomy, usually because it's something so new to them. As Mark Singer says: "My friends couldn't say ileitis or colitis, let alone know what it was like. But today they are getting an education because I'm speaking out and making others aware of the various aspects of ostomies."

Not everyone handles the situation that way. Some young adults prefer not to tell others about the ostomy. That's one nice thing about an ostomy: Because it's hidden, you can tell other people or not.

If any big problem arises—and stays big for quite a while—it's worth getting help. A teacher, or school counselor, or doctor, or an ET nurse may be able to help or may be able to suggest someone else who can help. Getting help for a big problem doesn't mean you've failed; it means instead that you are mature enough to know and use other resources.

Now many people having surgery for ulcerative colitis are having "alternative" procedures, such as an ileoanal anastomosis with reservoir. A reservoir procedure usually means a temporary ileostomy for a few weeks or months while the reservoir heals. Then there's another surgery, usually fairly minor, to get rid of the ileostomy and reconnect the intestine so that stool passes through the anus again. It often takes many months after that until the body learns to compensate for not having a colon anymore and the reservoir begins to function really well. Until then, although the ulcerative colitis is gone and the body can start feeling healthy again, there may still be frequent loose stools and sometimes leakage through the anus. It almost always gets better, much better, but it takes time.

Having patience during this period isn't easy for anyone, of any age. Talking to others who have gone through similar surgery can make it tolerable. The ET nurse, the surgeon, or the "Alternate Procedures" group from the United Ostomy Association (UOA) can steer you toward one person to talk to, or possibly a small group.

Some of the questions that young people with ostomies ask are ones older people ask too: How do I tell people? What about dates? What about sports? How about getting a job? Other chapters in this book talk about those subjects.

But there are some questions specific to teenagers. UOA sponsors an annual Youth Rally for young people ages 12 through 17 who have an ostomy, inflammatory bowel disease, an alternate procedure, or bowel or bladder incontinence. The event, several days of fun and learning held on a college campus or at a campground during the summer, combines new friendships, sports, crafts and social events with talks about everything from ostomy care to sexuality, drugs, and alcohol. For information, contact the United Ostomy Association, Inc., 36 Executive Park, Suite 120, Irvine, California, 92714-6744, Telephone 1-800-826-0826.

Some local UOA chapters have sub-groups for young people, or the regular UOA chapter may work out well for you. ET nurses are another resource for names of people who have gone through similar experiences. You are not alone, not the only one who has gone through this.

Nobody ever said it was easy to be a teenager.

When you're a teenager, the good times are not just good—they're incredible. But the bad times are so bleak that it's hard to believe there will ever be a good moment again. Adults may say, "Oh, it's going to get better. Stop mooning around and feeling sorry for yourself"—but that doesn't help at all.

All young people, with or without ostomies, face many of the same doubts, ask many of the same questions. Most are searching for independence; most are trying to live with bodies that are changing drastically and are frequently unpredictable. Most teenagers crave acceptance by other teenagers, and aren't always sure that they are accepted. Most wonder what they will do with their lives. Most are experiencing new feelings and sensations and relationships—and aren't too sure about any of it yet.

On the other hand, after an ostomy they may share the basic good health and high spirits common to young people. And they have a great capacity to make changes, to adapt to this slight change in the plumbing.

Talking with a friend, sharing good times and bad, seems to be one of the best ways to survive the teenage years. And when the questions and doubts are about an ostomy, the United Ostomy Association proves a faithful friend. As Marlene Vine puts it, it's "a one-to-one thing where someone has helped you, and you, in turn, help someone else."

CHAPTER 22 ❖ *Check-ups and Follow-ups*

*Being discharged from the hospital didn't mean
quite as much freedom as I'd hoped; the doctor
said to come back in two days.*

"Isn't it about time for your next appointment with the doctor?" my daughter asks.

"Maybe so. I'd better check." A foolish answer. I know the date better than my own birthday.

"How are you feeling?" she continues.

"Oh, fine." That's not quite true, either. Secretly I've written down a list of ten mysterious and probably dangerous symptoms to ask him about. And I'm working on number eleven.

We both know that somehow, just before a check-up, my medical imagination seems to go on a rampage. The tiniest symptom automatically means disaster, and I can see my entire intestinal tract coming apart as I wait.

In most cases, the actual check-up turns out to be a helpful, even comforting visit with a doctor I know and like. If there's a problem, it often gets a name. That makes it more manageable, and together we can search for a solution. After the appointment, I laugh at all that stupid, needless worry. I won't do that again. At least not until the next check-up. . .

For our friends who've had ileostomies to cure ulcerative colitis, surgery usually means the end of frequent and frustrating medical check-ups. After all, a nonexistent colon cannot become inflamed.

For most of the rest of us—whether the problem is Crohn's disease, cancer, or something else—regular check-ups are now a part of the game, although the time between medical appointments soon stretches. Every few days becomes once a month, then three months, six months, a year. If surgery was performed because of cancer, touching base regularly usually continues for the rest of one's life.

Much research, time and money have gone into the quest for an easy and sure test to identify cancer cells anywhere in the body, as accurately as a Geiger counter finds certain metals. Such a test would simplify early detection and thus multiply cures. It could also be used to follow-up patients who have been treated for cancer, both to check the success of any therapy and to detect any recurrence early so that it can be treated.

A move in that direction is a blood test for a "tumor marker" substance called *Carcino-embryonic Antigen* (CEA), often increased in the patient with colorectal cancer. If the CEA is above normal when the cancer is diagnosed, it returns to normal when the cancer is removed. The CEA blood test is then done periodically as part of the routine follow-up for colorectal cancer. Should the CEA rise again, more tests are performed to locate a possible recurrence.

For patients with either colorectal or bladder cancer, there's a push toward developing tests using *monoclonal antibodies* (MAbs), laboratory-grown copies of the protein produced by some of the body's defender cells. Like the body's own antibodies, MAbs "home in" on and attach themselves to "foreign" substances in the body (a particular kind of cancer cells, for instance). Large quantities of MAbs can be produced in the laboratory; then they can be tagged with a tiny bit of material which makes them show up on a special scan.

Injecting these tagged MAbs through the bloodstream so that perhaps they will "home in" on any hidden clusters of cancer cells is a technique sometimes tried now before ostomy surgery to guide the surgeon. Too, there is hope that, before long, this MAbs technology will provide a safe, easy, very accurate and relatively inexpensive test that could be done during follow-up visits to show if there are cancer cells present which need to be treated.

For now, doctors vary in the checks they make and the tests they order. Along with my list of ten scary questions (and a pad and pen for jotting down answers), I soon learned to take along a spare pouch in case the doctor wanted to examine my stoma. At least at first, stoma and perineal wound (if there is one) are frequently inspected. Weight is checked, along with blood and urine. Those who have urostomies will probably have IVPs as part of their ritual. If the ostomy surgery was performed for cancer, periodic pelvic and abdominal CT scans and chest x-rays are common tests.

(For the person with an ostomy who has had rectum and anus removed in an A-P resection, the doctor can no longer check a man's prostate gland or a woman's reproductive organs through the rectum as part of a routine physical exam. If there's a suspicion of a problem, other tests are necessary.)

People who have colostomies occasionally may undergo barium enema x-rays with the barium inserted through the stoma. Some x-ray staffs understand colostomies; many do not. The patient may need to use a little polite, informed assertiveness.

Having a colostomy may make a difference in the kind of bowel preparation necessary before the x-rays, so it is important to inform the staff when getting instructions for the "prep." The "prep"—which clears the bowel so that it can be seen well on x-ray—can involve a liquid diet and/or laxatives for a day or two before the test; a drainable pouch should be worn during this period. Some x-ray departments accept irrigation just before the barium enema as an adequate substitute for the usual laxatives. If there is more than one stoma or if the rectum and anus are still in place, enemas or irrigations through these openings may be ordered. For the x-rays, many people, whether they irrigate or not, take along an irrigation set or at least an irrigation cone to be slipped on the tube carrying the barium. Or, instead of a cone, a soft Foley catheter can be used; this has an inflatable balloon on it so that the barium stays inside the stoma.

Whether a cone or a Foley is used, it should be lubricated with surgical jelly and inserted gently but firmly into the stoma, preferably *by the patient.* To keep the barium in, the cone must be held firmly in place until the test is over. An irrigating sleeve will help control the barium, which wants to spurt all over the room the second the cone is removed.

Although some of the barium will splash out immediately, some will remain. Even when it is possible to irrigate immediately afterward in a nearby bathroom, it's prudent to wear a pouch home. More than one person, released from x-ray with a gut still partly full of barium and no appliance, has whitewashed his clothes and painted a pinkish-white stripe from front door to bathroom.

The opposite problem which can arise with barium is severe constipation. As the water which keeps the barium in suspension is absorbed by the colon, the insoluble barium hardens in the intestine. It's wise to irrigate as soon as possible afterward, or to take an approved laxative. Abundant warm fluids and food (especially items with a good percentage of fiber) also help prevent barium blockage.

During the last few years, most doctors have begun to substitute colonoscopy through the stoma for the barium enema. After the bowel is emptied, with the same preparation as for the barium enema, the doctor inspects the colon through the flexible lighted tube; pieces of tissue for biopsy can be removed, if necessary. Some medicine to relax the person is given before the procedure.

As surgical techniques have improved, the need to revise stomas has decreased. Occasionally, scar tissue causes blockage and must be removed. If a stoma *retracts* (draws in) or *prolapses* (protrudes) farther than it should, causing management problems, surgical correction may be necessary. Sometimes a person with an ostomy can get a *hernia* around the stoma. In most cases, the problem is not severe enough to require surgery and wearing a wide support ostomy belt is sufficient, but sometimes, surgical revision is preferable to suffering long-term pouching difficulties.

For the person with a temporary ostomy, it sometimes takes many check-ups before it's time to reconnect the intestine (and do away with the stoma). Months or even years may pass before everything is right for the switch back. The reasons for such procedures are so varied that there can be no general rules. In many cases, although the surgery is major, reconnection is easier than the operation which created the temporary ostomy. For one thing, the individual is apt to be in far better health. For another, there are few surprises when one knows what to expect. Once in a while, there's a surprising twinge of doubt: The ostomy's working so well—why not just leave it alone?

On any trip to the hospital (whether to have a baby, a stoma revised, or an ingrown toenail removed), the person with an ostomy may need to help educate hospital staff, especially on nonsurgical floors where such patients may be rare birds. The person can bring along two cards with basic information on them, one to give to the admitting nurse so that facts can be recorded on the nursing summary (where basic information about the patient is kept), the other to display prominently on the bedside table. As an example, a person with an ileostomy who has had her rectum removed might include this information: *ATTENTION: Patient has an ileostomy. Do not take rectal temperature. Do not give enemas. Do not give laxatives. Do not irrigate ileostomy. Do not remove pouch from abdomen.* Even with these cards, the patient may have to speak up loudly—if a nurse approaches with a rectal thermometer.

Since not all hospitals know that Joe Blow's Velvet Touch Pouches are the best in the world, people who have had their ostomies for a while learn to bring their own supplies, including an irrigation set with irrigation sleeves if used and, for the sake of staff and roommates, a supply of a pouch deodorant or satisfactory room deodorizer. An IV pole can hold the irrigation bag, but is too high; strong twine or a wire coat hanger bent so there is a hook at each end solves the problem. Many people choose to forget irrigating if they're bed-bound. Once they're up and around again, they can get back on schedule with little trouble. In the meantime, disposable drainable pouches allow them freedom to concentrate on getting well.

When ostomy surgery is performed because of cancer, the doctor may recommend radiation, chemotherapy, and/or biological therapy to increase the effectiveness of the surgery. Radiation can further shrink tumors and destroy any cancer cells still lurking in the immediate area. Chemotherapy uses powerful drugs to combat stray cancer cells anywhere in the body. Biological therapy stimulates the body's own defense system so it will recognize and destroy cancer cells wherever they are.

All these therapies are potent medicine, offering many possible benefits and, sometimes, unpleasant side effects.

Radiation, which may be done before, after, or even during surgery, involves a carefully-planned series of treatments. The radiation therapist aims the powerful beam at the cancer site, where it will do the most good, and carefully shields other areas so the tissues will not be damaged. The patient usually comes to the radiation department every day, often for a few weeks, and lies on a table for the brief, painless treatment. The person is *not* radioactive.

Since radiation treatments destroy not only cancer cells but also some normal cells in the beam's field, the therapy can cause temporary fatigue as the body works overtime to repair damaged tissues. Temporary skin redness (like sunburn) often develops in the area being treated. Depending on the radiation field, a person may develop some nausea, diarrhea, or urinary complaints which can often be helped by medication. Occasionally, side effects appear after the therapy is over.

Any external ostomy pouch is removed if radiation is given to the area of the stoma. The radiation therapy staff or an ET nurse can give instructions about what ostomy products can be used safely on the skin during the weeks of treatment. The person with a colostomy who irrigates often needs to wear a pouch during the weeks of treatment and for some time afterwards because of temporary loose stools.

Chemotherapy has brought about dramatic improvements and cures with some kinds of cancer. In others, it is still at the experimental stage. Most of the drugs used work best on cells which divide quickly, including those in some bladder cancers. Until recently, chemotherapy was much less effective with colorectal cancer, but new regimens (often combining both chemotherapy and biological therapy drugs) have shown considerable promise.

The fast-dividing cells which chemotherapy drugs attack include not only cancer cells but also such healthy cells as the blood-making cells in the bone marrow, the cells lining the digestive tract, and hair cells. However, while the cancer cells die, the normal cells recover: That's what makes chemotherapy work.

Some people have few symptoms, but many report fatigue, nausea, hair loss, or other problems. Some symptoms can be prevented or treated during therapy, and most are reversible after the therapy finishes.

Chemotherapy drugs are given through a vein or artery, by mouth, by injection into the muscle, into the bladder, or by other routes. Two or more drugs which work in different ways are often combined for greater effectiveness against the cancer cells and fewer side effects.

Many intravenous chemotherapy drugs can be given in the doctor's office; others require periodic short hospital stays. Some people receive their "chemo" continuously through a vein by way of a small pump. These ambulatory pumps, the size of a deck of cards or smaller, are either worn next to the body or implanted under the skin—and allow people to go about their normal business during treatment. The pumps can be refilled at the doctor's office; the implanted pumps are "accessed" for refilling with a needle through the skin.

Biological therapy is the newcomer in cancer treatment. It's not new at all in treating other diseases, since every vaccination against measles or polio follows a basic biological therapy strategy: teaching the body's own immune cells to attack something which shouldn't be there.

The body's own defenses, which recognize obvious invaders like bacteria, have a harder time with cancer cells, which aren't as unmistakably foreign. Biological therapy uses highly-purified proteins to wake up the body's defenses or make them work together better. Or it tries to increase the numbers of defender cells, make the individual cells more effective, or mark the cancer cells more clearly as targets.

Biological therapies for bladder and/or colorectal cancer may include injections of proteins (like interferons or interleukins) that increase communication among the immune cells. Colony-stimulating factors can speed the growth of large numbers of defender cells, if these have been decreased by other cancer therapy. Monoclonal antibodies may be able to attach themselves to cancer cells and alert the body's defenses to attack; if the monoclonal antibodies have a payload of chemotherapy drugs or radioactive material, they may act as "smart bombs" to destroy cancer cells. Or BCG vaccine, used originally for tuberculosis and now used for some bladder cancers, may be able to activate the immune system to produce its own antibodies. These biological therapy agents are injected through a vein, into a muscle or under the skin, placed in the bladder, or given by other routes.

Promising as biological therapies are, there are still problems when it comes to using them for colorectal or bladder cancers. The monoclonal antibodies may target the wrong cells, for instance, or the body may start seeing the biological therapy proteins as foreign and attack them. As with chemotherapy or radiation, side effects occasionally can make the patient miserable, or can even be life-threatening.

None of these treatments (radiation, chemotherapy, or biological therapy) should be undertaken lightly. Specific information is available from the cancer specialists—the medical and radiation *oncologists.*

As always, the wise patient becomes a real member of the treatment team. This means asking questions, gathering information in words one can understand, and talking over concerns with the doctor. It means learning about the potential benefits and possible problems of all the therapy options (including no treatment) before making choices *with* the doctor. A second opinion may be helpful.

While it's crucial that the oncologist be knowledgeable and skilled, it's also important that he or she be a person one can talk with, honestly and comfortably. Among the oncologist's many jobs is laying to rest some of the "old wives' tales" about cancer and its therapies. With new medications and techniques to prevent or lessen side effects, cancer treatment can be powerful and tolerable at the same time.

Tumor boards, groups of cancer specialists who meet to discuss treatment choices for individual patients with cancer, can guide the patient. It's also a good idea to check with a large cancer center and/or with the Cancer Information Service of the National Cancer Institute (telephone: 1-800-4-CANCER) about new options.

Clinical trials, which test a new therapy or combination of therapies under stringent conditions, may be available for patients with colorectal or bladder cancer. These experimental treatments are tried because there is a reasonable hope that they will be more effective than current therapies; they can be the source of treatment breakthroughs. Clinical trials often involve one group of patients receiving the experimental treatment and a second "control" (comparison) group receiving the standard treatment.

With any of these treatments, attitude is important. Emotional support, medication to offset side effects, relaxation techniques, and interesting diversion are all part of the program. Tempting and nutritious food is an essential ally.

For most people with ostomies, ET nurses suggest regular appointments during the first year and recommend checking in once in a while after that. There may be a new pouch which will solve a lot of problems; weight gains may have changed the kind or size of appliance needed. Often, little tiny problems never get a chance to grow large if they're spotted when they're small.

In a novel, *To Build A Ship*, Don Berry has something to say about survival: "Man is by nature a victim. But when he knows he can survive anything—he rebels, and is no longer a victim. He feels the power of his own surviving in his belly and it makes him wake up in the middle of the night and turn under his blankets with a secret smile. For the first time he realizes there is more to living than merely submitting. . . ."

Check-ups are one of the resources that help us feel the power of our own surviving, and turn under our blankets with a secret smile. . .

CHAPTER 23 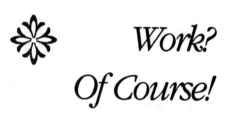 *Work?*
Of Course!

> *Work—keep everlasting at it, for it is*
> *the darlingest gift of the gods.*
> Mark Twain

There are times, like the Monday morning commute rush, when our zeal for work may not match Twain's. But satisfying work is a blessing (and pays the bills), and an ostomy seldom prevents an individual from finding or keeping a job.

If the firsthand accounts of thousands of doctors, stenographers, truck drivers, housewives, salespeople, nurses, teachers, bricklayers, professional athletes, musicians, mailmen, volunteers, scientists, plumbers, mechanics, policemen, and others mean anything, people with ostomies do just about everything—and do it well. Every time someone suggests an occupation which a person with an ostomy "just can't do," someone else has on the tip of the tongue the account of a friend with an ostomy who has that job. It used to be taken as gospel that people with ostomies could be anything—except belly dancers or professional football players. Then a belly dancer and a professional football player with ostomies turned up.

It's a third-hand tale, but one friend insists that a San Francisco Bay Area doctor has a patient who worked in a rodeo; after ostomy surgery, the doctor told the patient he could return to his job. "Later he found out the patient rides Brahma bulls and so the doctor asked the man if it didn't create a problem. The patient said: 'Yeah, I lost my bag but I didn't mind, the bull didn't mind, and I won anyway!'"

As Ed Gambrell, a past president of UOA, says flatly: "... an ostomy is not an illness. It is the fully manageable result of a procedure to *cure* an illness or to *remedy* a disorder."

Richard Daniels, a food chemist who has lived and worked with an ileostomy for over a quarter of a century, suggests four basic questions for anyone thinking of a job:

1. Am I physically able to do the job?

2. Will my employer take me back? (Or will this employer hire me?)

3. Will I be accepted by my fellow employees?

4. Will my changed bathroom habits cause any problems?

Am I physically able to do the job? Until the patient recovers from surgery and learns to live comfortably with the ostomy, the thought of lifting anything heavier than a toothbrush may be overwhelming. Even after full recovery from surgery, people have different levels of energy and strength to balance against the physical demands of a particular job. Most of the time, if the person with the ostomy really wants *that* job, there is a way to make it possible.

The person thinking about a job requiring very heavy lifting, for instance, may find it sufficient to wear a sturdy support garment and to review the best ways to lift heavy objects—or he may want to set his sights on a job without such heavy lifting. In a very hot job, like on the fire line of an aluminum plant, the person with an ileostomy may need to consume an electrolyte-rich "sports" drink by the gallon to ward off dehydration. A comfortable cushion can ease the twinges of a still tender perineal wound for someone who drives a bus.

Will my employer take me back? Or will this employer hire me? These questions don't arise at all for the self-employed. The lawyer, the housewife, the artist, the store owner can return to the job without breaking step. And many people with ostomies, their surgery time covered by accumulated sick leave, rejoin their company without a ripple of a problem.

Others may find a few obstacles on the path. If the employer has an opening, and if the person with an ostomy has the experience, ability and desire to fill that opening, the employer still can have some reasonable questions: What is the past work and absenteeism record? What is the prognosis for this person after this kind of surgery? Is this employment going to create any special problems for me, the employer?

A personal physician or the medical adviser of the local UOA chapter can smooth the way. If absenteeism before surgery was a problem—very common if inflammatory bowel disease led to the ostomy—the doctor can reassure the employer: The ostomy should decrease the absences. Questions about prognosis too can be answered in a phone call or letter from the physician.

Some employers balk at hiring or rehiring the person with an ostomy because they don't know much about ostomies and it's easier just to say "no." What people with ostomies take for granted is completely foreign to some employers who may not even know what an ostomy *is*, let alone that a person can live a normal, comfortable, productive life with one. Some basic information and gentle assertiveness by both jobseeker and physician can topple old prejudices and can answer specific questions about such matters as company insurance, physical ability, or worker's compensation. After all, as Ed Gambrell points out, "an ostomate's employability should be given thoughtful and fair consideration, not just on behalf of the ostomate who may already be employed or who is looking for a job, but also in the interest of the employer who seeks to hire and retain good employees."

Will I be accepted by my fellow employees? *If the person accepts the ostomy, others will too.* Doing the job and treating others with consideration (leaving the bathroom clean and odor-free, for instance) are essential. Whether or not to tell fellow employees about an ostomy is a personal choice; since the ostomy is invisible under work clothes, no one will know unless one wishes to tell. Many people hesitate to tell others until they are well established in a job, and then tell one or two friends. Others share their experiences more readily.

Will my changed bathroom habits cause any problems? It is more comfortable to have access to a convenient bathroom. If pouches need frequent drainage or expulsion of air, the employee and the supervisor may need to arrange for a desk closer to the bathroom or perhaps for shorter, more frequent "coffee breaks." The right to this type of "accommodation" is provided in the U.S. under the Disabilities Act of 1990.

Many people—students, women entering the job market after staying home with a family—apply for their first paid job after an ostomy. A shaky job market and lack of employment experience cause far more problems than the ostomy. School counselors, Department of Employment counselors, classes on getting a job all can help.

Other people with ostomies change jobs after surgery. Some choose new careers in the health field—sometimes as doctors or nurses or ET nurses—as a direct result of their own experiences. Many reassess their priorities after surgery and decide to pursue a career they always wanted to follow but, for one reason or another, never did. Some find that the stress level of the pre-surgery job is unacceptable and find a job where there are fewer, or different, stressors. Some, freed for the first time in years from chronic bowel disease, explore the many new avenues open to them.

And some people just want a change, like Jim Holladay who turned from contracting to serious carpentry after his colostomy—at age 88!

For the person with an ostomy who cannot, for any good reason, return to a former occupation, sometimes the state department of rehabilitation can finance job retraining if the doctor recommends it. It's worth considering, if there's a problem.

One big question for people with ostomies who are seeking jobs is "How much do I tell the Personnel Office?" David Rightman of the Los Angeles Department of Employment wishes that more people would pioneer, volunteering full information to their prospective employers. That way, he contends, more employers would know about the excellent employees they have already and would be more willing to hire other people with ostomies.

But, when the current employment situation is tight, many people prefer to downplay the ostomy, perhaps informing the employer *after* a period of satisfactory employment. This does not mean lying or falsifying answers, of course. But as Ed Claitman, from Pittsburgh, counsels: "One question that continually comes up from many, many people applying for employment with corporations is under the heading of 'Do you have a physical handicap?' We consistently recommend that you answer 'NO,' as we do not consider an ostomy a handicap. If there is a question about surgery, within a specific time limit, obviously you must honestly answer that question. It boils down to the fact that unless the question is very, very specific, where to AVOID mentioning an ostomy is a false statement, then do nothing to bring it out."

When Mary St. John started looking for a job, she had a new ileostomy after five months of hospitalization for ulcerative colitis: "It was at that point that I first came up against the cruel, hard world. As far as I was concerned, I felt I was perfectly healthy and normal and in much better shape than many of my peers. But with this terrible medical history, I found that most companies were a little reluctant—and that is an understatement!—to have anything to do with an ostomate. I had a lot of doors slammed in my face and I was pretty unhappy about it." One of the things I did was apply at many of the companies that are government contractors, and they usually require security clearance. You have to go through this very involved rigamarole of filling out complicated forms, and there is always a little block about medical history. I was so candid and honest about this I think, perhaps, I was frightening some people. We are all very comfortable and relaxed about ostomy surgery, but for people who are not familiar with this sort of thing it is a shock, and they are sometimes taken up short by it.

"I finally made up a little plan. I don't like to think of this as dishonest. I'd like to think it is one of those sins of omission. When I would come to the little spot in the application which said, 'Have you ever had serious illness or surgery?' I would say, 'Yes, in 1964 I had an intestinal infection. The condition was surgically cured by removal of the infected section of the intestine.' And that was that. I was finally employed by a very well-known company which I stayed with for about two and a half years. Two months ago, I left it and went to work for my present employer. He knew about my ileostomy, but I had to fill out the form and take a physical. So I hied myself off to the handy dandy little company physician and went through the whole chest thumping thing. He looked at my form and said, 'Well, now Miss St. John, I see you've had some surgery. How is your colitis?'

"'Just fine, it never bothers me. I no longer have a colon, so I don't have much trouble with colitis,' and that was the end of that!"

Most people with ostomies who want a job and are otherwise qualified get a job eventually, although there may be missteps along the way—which one can laugh at, *later*. Don Binder, former Executive Director of UOA and a commercial artist, was refused when he applied for his first job after surgery: ". . .the examining physician kept calling my ileostomy a colostomy. I couldn't understand how a doctor could confuse the two when I knew well the difference."

The more personal elements of job-seeking and keeping—liking oneself, ostomy and all, and communicating that good self-image to employer and other employees—come easily to some people, less easily to others. Talking to other people with ostomies who have jobs can help. Concentrating on the job to be done rather than on oneself can carry one smoothly through the job application process and those first few days of work.

There are several other strategies for the job-seeker. If there are gaps in employment because of illness or treatment, the resume can downplay this if it's organized by skills and achievements rather than chronologically by dates of employment

It isn't necessary to volunteer any information about health history (although any direct questions must be answered honestly). However, one can qualify any "yes" to a question about health history in an application or interview with positive statements about current health. Often it helps to practice answering possible questions before a job interview—getting used to projecting a confident rather than a defensive attitude.

What if the person with an ostomy applies for a specific opening for which he or she is well qualified, takes care with the job interview (comes on time, neatly dressed and so on), answers satisfactorily any questions about past absenteeism, current prognosis, physical ability, (with the help of the personal physician or the medical advisor of the local UOA chapter, if necessary)—and still doesn't get the job, apparently because of the ostomy? What then?

In the U.S., the right of the person with an ostomy to work is protected to some extent by the *US Rehabilitation Act of 1973* and the *Americans with Disabilities Act of 1990*. Many U.S. employers are prohibited from basing hiring decisions on what are *perceived* to be disability conditions. Sections of state and provincial (in Canada) laws also apply. Federal and state agencies enforce and give information about these laws. The UOA is a resource; if the ostomy is cancer-related, the American (or Canadian) Cancer Society may be able to help. An attorney with experience in resolving job discrimination problems is a possibility, although other avenues should be exhausted first.

If cancer led to the ostomy, the National Coalition for Cancer Survivorship provides a periodic newsletter as well as packets of information about both job and insurance discrimination against cancer patients. NCCS can be reached at 1010 Wayne Avenue, 5th Floor, Silver Spring, MD 20910, telephone (301) 585-2616. The National Cancer Institute (NCI) of the U.S. Department of Health and Human Services issues a free pamphlet, *Facing Forward: A Guide for Cancer Survivors*, which addresses employment and insurance questions; the booklet is available by phone from the Cancer Information Service at 1-800-4-CANCER.

Insurance remains a thorny issue for many people who have undergone ostomy surgery, whether because of cancer, inflammatory bowel disease or another problem. Sometimes people have major difficulty obtaining health insurance or getting their insurance company to cover expenses. Another major problem is that many people feel trapped in the wrong job because they are afraid of losing insurance coverage if they leave, or of getting insurance which won't cover a preexisting condition.

This isn't a problem in countries which have national health insurance. In the U.S., federal or state governments cover basic health care for some groups of people: Most people 65 or older and the permanently disabled (Medicare); some people who are unemployed or in low-income brackets (Medicaid, called Medi-Cal in California); and some veterans (VA medical centers).

Other options, besides a regular company plan for the employed person with an ostomy, include: dependent coverage under a spouse's insurance plan; a health maintenance organization (HMO) with an open enrollment period in which a person must be accepted regardless of health history; group insurance through a professional, fraternal or other organization to which the person belongs.

Some states offer "high risk" health insurance pools for people who can't get insurance any other way; current information on these is available from the UOA headquarters office (1-800-826-0826). The "Blues" (Blue Cross and Blue Shield) have open enrollment periods in some states. A few independent insurance brokers are experts at matching people with some form of health insurance, although the coverage may have high deductibles and limited coverage. Both the Crohn's and Colitis Foundation of America, Inc. and the UOA national organization have made the insurability issue a priority—and hope to see results of their efforts soon.

This insurance picture could change in the U.S. at any time as the federal government and the states investigate different ways of paying for the health needs of citizens. People everywhere are showing all kinds of employers that an ostomy is no bar to employment. TV programs, newspaper stories, service club programs all spread the word. But individuals working well in individual jobs spread the word most effectively.

When Linda Schwartz graduated from the University of Southern California School of Pharmacy, she was hired as one of the full-time pharmacists—at the hospital where she had had her ostomy surgery at the age of six.

Or there's Horace Saunders, who continues to work at his chosen profession as a custom tailor with a clientele that includes movie stars and senators.

Or Marilou Tinay who returned to her job as an airline flight attendant after a complete jejunostomy (leaving only 13 inches, or 33 cm, of small intestine) for Crohn's disease—and runs an ostomy supply store in her "spare" time.

Or there's. . .

CHAPTER 24 ❊ *Swimming, Skiing and Other Diversions*

*Although I'll never be quite as eager a sports person as my friend Carol Norris, I can't blame my inertia on my ostomy. Carol, on the other hand, is a runner, **thanks** to her ileostomy. Before that happened, she says, she was a Florida-grown indoor type who preferred curling up with a book to running.*

The way Carol tells it, "After my ulcerative colitis ileostomy at 27, I hiked, but preferably downhill, and without a back-pack. At 38 I began jogging, and at 40 I'd reached three miles, three times a week. That is the turning point for easily doubling distances. My husband shamed me by reaching marathon-running in his first six months, while I kept coming in last at club races of 2-5 miles. When a boy of 4 and woman of 70 ran in our local marathon, I decided to train harder. Now I've run two half-marathons (13.1 miles each) and hope someday to better that distance." (She did, completing the Helinski marathon.)

Since people with ostomies are people first, their reasons for choosing any physical activity are basically those of anyone else: to feel good, to be healthy, and to enjoy the activity. As Carol pinpoints it, "How I regret the lazy years when I did no jogging, when I had to watch my diet, enlarge my clothes, and gasp on one flight of stairs. . . .Let your body assert itself and find health. Hit the road, sisters!"

An ostomy is certainly no hindrance to sports of all kinds—running, jogging, swimming, sailing, skiing, bowling, golf, bicycling and tennis, to name a few. Babe Didrickson Zaharias won the U.S. Women's Open Golf Championship in 1954, after her colostomy for cancer in 1953. People with ostomies participate as gymnasts, fencers, football players, sky divers, skin divers, and hockey players. Name the sport and there are people with ostomies involved, playing hard, with no limit on their enjoyment.

Even the simplest exercise does wonders for getting and keeping abdominal muscles firm, and appetite and digestive tract in good order. Swimming and walking are among the best. In the months just after surgery, this may mean sauntering instead of an extended hike, or only a lap or two of a swimming pool instead of twenty. Whatever kind it is, activity speeds healing.

Before surgery, I'd enjoyed the pool in the courtyard almost daily, so I was eager to return to swimming, especially during the hot August days. After checking with my doctor, I cautiously and rather self-consciously edged down the pool steps, picking a time when the pool was almost deserted. My legs had as much power as two soggy strands of spaghetti—they wouldn't kick. Besides, I was worrying about my pouch leaking or showing. Even so, the water felt wonderful, lapping my body, soothing yet invigorating. Maybe I was getting well—except for those lazy legs.

A few hints before I tried the pool could have increased my confidence—and pleasure. If I'd known abdominal muscles (which have a lot to do with controlling leg movements) almost always take time to regain their tone after major surgery, I'd have been less upset by temporarily-wilted legs. And if I'd tried reading in the bathtub for an hour or so, complete with pouch and bathing suit, before trying the pool, I wouldn't have worried about appliance security.

There are other common-sense tips for swimmers who wear a pouch. If a belt is used, it should be rubber or nylon, perhaps worn a little more snugly than usual; elastic belts stretch when wet. A picture frame of waterproof tape will hold most appliances securely. Although skin barriers are not generally exposed to water, karaya is water-soluble; to be completely safe, other choices may be better for swimming. A thin panty girdle or jockey-type shorts may be worn under a swimsuit or men's swimming briefs. Style depends not only on stoma location but on personal preference—and current fashion. There are bikini wearers among women with ostomies, but many feel more comfortable with one-piece suits (albeit with plunging necklines), and some like suits with a skirt, or belted shift styles. For the person with a sigmoid colostomy, a "colostomy plug" is an option.

Anyone with a new ostomy needs to take it easy at first. There is the recent surgery to recover from, one day at a time. Many, too, are free for the first time in years from an illness which kept them sedentary and thus out of condition.

Even those in superb condition before surgery, like Otto Graham, captain, U.S. Coast Guard Academy, and former professional football star with the Cleveland Browns, may find it necessary to go slow at first. Graham discovered that being forced to try a slower pace had a real, if unexpected, benefit. An active tennis player and golfer before surgery, he believes his games are ". . .as good if not better than they were before my operation.

"In golf, I was so weak at first I had to swing very slowly and let the club do the work. As everyone knows, this is the best way to swing a golf club; swing easy and let the club do the work. And this has carried over, even though I have regained my strength."

Teenage hockey player Richard Alperin, of Holbrook, Massachusetts, rebelled at taking it easy at first and started playing ice hockey two short months after his continent ileostomy. This didn't give his new internal pouch enough time to heal securely. But five months after a second surgery, Richard was back on the ice, this time with no ill effects. After he received his high school diploma and started working he wrote: "I get a lot of exercise and wouldn't consider working at a job which wasn't physical. . . .I'm a very active person and enjoy getting completely exhausted."

Evan Deutsch, of Southfield, Michigan, began running marathons after ostomy surgery. After gaining 50 pounds in the two months following his ileostomy, he decided the most enjoyable way to stay lean—was to run.

Aside from the pleasure of participating, and the good things physical activity does for one's general health, people with ostomies know that sports heal mind as well as body. Exercise remains one of the best ways around for dealing with anger, depression, worry, and increased tensions, problems that may decrease a person's resistance to disease. Physical activity, by providing an outlet for stress, is one of the best medicines available.

Runner Michael Komlos sets himself a goal of 3000 miles a year. "I remember when I first started to run I was really out of breath. I came back home after running two miles and laid down on the kitchen floor. I thought I was going to die. But after a short rest, I went right back outside and started to run again."

Michael claims that he runs for health, but "just as importantly, I run for my spiritual and mental well being.

"I can really be alone with my thoughts when I'm running. It's just a total release."

People with ostomies also point to the confidence they get with sports. Self-image problems (often enormous right after the surgery) recede as they are able to say to themselves, "Look what I can do!"

Lori Musser, a gymnast from Tucson, Arizona, had her ileostomy when she was 11, after a two-year bout with colitis. As she tells it, "I started my freshman year in high school on the tennis team. I wasn't much of a tennis player, but with a lot of practice, I got to where I could get the ball over the net (part of the time!). I was at the bottom of the ladder most of the time, it was something I was accustomed to because, before my surgery, I never *felt* like trying anything, so of course I didn't do well in anything. But this time it didn't bother me because I was trying. . . .

"The chance to try has been very important to me. I've seen so many people who say 'I can't' when they haven't even tried. Maybe their reasons are good, but if it's the fear of defeat, that isn't good. You can't open yourself to the chance for a victory without the possibility of defeat.

"At the end of my freshman year, I tried out for cheerleading and. . .made it! There I was, probably the shyest person at school, and for two years I jumped around in front of a crowd like I honestly belonged there. . . .I must admit. . .there were a few times when a lot of tape eased a few worries.

"I've been in gymnastics now for four years. . . .I'd seen Cathy Rigby whipping around those bars and I wasn't so sure how well my stoma was going to like that. I told my coach I had an ileostomy and I didn't know if there would be any trouble or not. She said, simply, 'That's okay, just don't do anything that gives you trouble.'

"...Well, I'm no great gymnast, there are a lot of things I can't do, but there's nothing I can't do because of my stoma. . . .

"Besides a strong love for the excitement of being a gymnast, it's those strangers whom I came to know and love after my surgery, the ones who said, 'You can, Lori, You can!' And the fact that I can *try*. I fall and come home with new bruises all the time, but I can try!

"As far as my stoma is concerned, well, without it, I wouldn't have those voices implanted in my mind that drive me to higher goals. And more important than that, I wouldn't be alive to try."

Sports offer something for everyone: for the person who prefers gentle exercise in private and for those who like the companionship of shared sports, competitive or noncompetitive. There's a sport for everyone—from miniature golf to skin diving.

Barbara Hurewitz of the Ileostomy Association of New York had always wanted to try fencing, but her chance didn't come until after her ileostomy: "I was worried at first about the idea of a sword piercing my appliance, but this proved to be an imaginary fear. If you wear a long fencing jacket or even a sweater, you are more than adequately protected against a fencing foil."

Barbara also recommends dancing as a sport but warns beginning dancers to go easy on abdominal stretches and exercises at first. For dancers, she suggests a dance tunic or a short dance skirt over a leotard for women, a short tunic over briefs for men.

Belly dancing used to be called 'the only activity closed to people with ostomies,' but Jo Madsen of Eureka, California—who also happens to be a grandmother—belly dances for special events. She also practices yoga, runs two miles a day, and swims as often as she can. As a frequent traveler, she often startles flight attendants when she continues her habit of daily headstands even on the airplane, sometimes in the aisle!

Ellen P. Fincher of Orange County, a born athlete, joyously started horseback riding at 13 but was soon stopped by a long two-year fight with ulcerative colitis. However, within a year after her surgery she was riding again, and also found time to get married and find a job. Now she and her husband participate in equestrian events three weekends a month, saving the fourth for meetings of the Orange County Ostomy Association!

Most people with ostomies have no special problems skiing. One who does—but has found ways to overcome them—is Larry Kunz of Colorado. Born with a severe spinal defect, Larry can barely walk and has minimal control of his legs and feet. He had a urostomy when he was six years old. After moving to Colorado from New York, he took up skiing. His instructor, Hal O'Leary, had established a special ski program for people with physical disabilities, but had never taught anyone with *spina bifida*. Excited at first, Larry became discouraged:

"It was really, really tough. But then one day, Hal started yelling at me, 'Do you want to be a cripple all your life?'

"That was the turning point."

Now Larry can ski any slope, any sort of terrain. He uses "outriggers," crutch-like devices with ski bottoms, instead of conventional poles, and he schusses the slopes with the tips of his skis tied together by a six-inch length of nylon.

"That's to keep me from doing the splits and hurting myself," explains Larry. "And if I'm going to race, I tie them even closer together."

For anyone contemplating a return to or a first try at a sport, there are a few common-sense reminders:

Check with your doctor first. He or she can advise you

on any limitations imposed either by your surgery or your general condition.

Pick a sport that sounds like fun to you. If all your friends are jogging but you loathe the idea, try something else. Bernice Kaufman Ordover advises that "Exercise should be relaxing, comfortable and fun!. . .Most people put themselves into a rigid exercise program, get sore muscles and give it up. They punish themselves and then their body rejects it. Try dancing at home to your favorite music. Jog when you walk the dog. Use your legs and not the wheels of your car."

Take it easy at first. Getting utterly exhausted during your first session will only make you discouraged and unnecessarily sore. Building muscles and endurance slowly works better for any prospective athlete, with or without an ostomy.

Use the right equipment. This goes not only for equipment specific for each sport—like comfortable jogging shoes for joggers or proper protective equipment for football players—but for ostomy equipment as well. Security during active movement is your goal. A little trial and error plus some advice from other sports-minded people with ostomies can help. You may want to switch from your regular equipment, perhaps add a belt, try a panty girdle or close-fitting jockey shorts. All that activity, heat, and perspiration may make more frequent pouch changes necessary. And it makes sense to start out with an empty appliance. Don't forget to replace all those fluids lost in perspiration. After all, the electrolyte-rich "sports" drinks were developed for athletes.

Physical Education major Karen Koehler, from New York, includes softball, basketball, volleyball, hockey, golf, archery, badminton and tennis in her college regimen. Her ostomy did cause her a problem once. In the third quarter of an "away" basketball game (with her team a few points behind) vigorous play plus a collision with an opponent caused her appliance to loosen. Quickly she asked the referee to excuse her from the game for medical reasons, dashed to the locker room, and used her emergency kit. She was back in the game in time for the fourth quarter—and in time to score the winning three points!

Keep playing. It takes time for all the benefits of a sport to show. Regular exercise pays far more dividends in terms of health, looks, and energy than intense sporadic spurts, alternating with bouts of inertia.

Most of all, *enjoy it.*

What gymnast Lori Musser says is worth repeating: ". . .There are a lot of things I can't do, but there's nothing I can't do because of my stoma. . . ."

CHAPTER 25   ✧ *The Other Side of the World*

After surgery, they think they're never going to be able to travel again, not even from San Francisco to Colma, just twenty miles away! Then pretty soon—maybe six months later—I get a beautiful picture postcard from this patient, saying "Wish you were here," and it's postmarked Tokyo or someplace else—they're off on a 45-day cruise!
(From a conversation with Jean Alvers, ET, San Francisco)

Far from stopping people from traveling, ostomies seem to act as mysterious catalysts that send them on their way! People with ostomies go *everywhere:* from backpacking in the Sierra to grand tours of Europe, traveling by foot, bicycle, horseback, car, boat, plane, roller skates, and camelback.

Many of us take that scary first trip after surgery just to prove it can be done. Then, bitten by the travel bug, some of us keep on going. This is an exciting world, and many people, whether freed from misery for the first time in years, or given a new chance at life (and some new priorities for living) want to see it all.

Perhaps not *everyone* is as adventurous as Esther E. Komarend of Boston. "I went 'Around the World in 68 Days.' I visited 17 countries, flew 19,600 air miles on 29 airplanes, rode on an elephant and camel, glided in a canoe over rapids, found myself on dugouts, sampans, junks, walked about 140 miles, climbed hundreds of stairs, and enjoyed all the excitement that went with all of it. . . After suffering from ulcerative colitis for twelve years, the ileostomy surgery I so dreaded has really made my life more beautiful. . . .Where next?"

Burt and Thelma Blanchard of Glendale, California, use ten-speed bikes instead of airplanes or elephants (although they fly or take the train to their take-off point). On bikes, they followed the 1804-1806 Lewis and Clark Trail for some 600 miles from Missoula, Montana, to Portland, Oregon.

After Burt's ileostomy surgery in 1964, and recovery from a major heart attack in 1972, the Blanchards knew they needed regular exercise and, with the doctor's approval, chose biking. Beginning with short rides around the neighborhood, they started reaching out with more miles and overnight trips. A few years later, this over-fifty couple enjoyed a two-week biking vacation, exploring the San Juan Islands of Puget Sound. That convinced them that "as long as we were well prepared, we could handle just about any kind of bike tour." Inspired by success, they began training for that Lewis and Clark Trail ride.

It makes sense to wait until you've bounced back from surgery, and are reasonably comfortable with your ostomy, before setting out. To gain confidence, many people suggest short trips first. For instance, George A. McConney of Kalamazoo, Michigan, reports:

"When my urostomy was six months old, I took it to Chicago for an overnight stay. How simple that sounds, but how far from simple it was to me at that time!. . .The thought of going far away from my own bathroom, and sleeping in a strange bed was frightening. I packed enough equipment to last me for two weeks and we set out.

"With beginner's luck, nothing happened!" After completing his business, there was time for sightseeing, and for reflection: "Probably nothing before or since has done more to reconcile me to my urostomy than this trip without any problems."

After a similar dry run, the world's your oyster. . .

Inspired by the overnight trip to Chicago, the McConneys decided they not only could travel but must:

"Surviving these difficulties, we tramped the streets of Rome, Florence, Venice and Naples and had a wonderful time. It was kind of a honeymoon. . .I came home feeling that I could do anything I had done before my operation.

"The period that followed our return home was a tremendous letdown. Bags came unstuck day and night. This produced a general demoralization. It was also a period of particular stress at work. I began to feel that I could only function properly when on vacation!"

Acting on this intuition, the McConneys have since gone across the U.S., to Mexico, British Columbia, Central America, Greece and Turkey.

Other people with ostomies and ET nurses delight in sharing travel tips, along with their photographs and suntans. Here are some favorites:

First, *have a wonderful time!* You may face a few new challenges (as most travelers do) but, if you pack your sense of humor along with other necessities, they won't stop you.

Think ahead. Before you go, picture (as well as you can) the places you'll be and plan for privacy and security. For instance, one woman we know and her husband planned a cross-country drive to visit relatives who had a large house, a large family and just one bathroom. She decided to forget irrigating until she got home. Instead, she took along a good supply of disposable pouches so she wouldn't have to worry about any time limits on privacy.

Get any prescriptions needed—or recommendations for non-prescription drugs. Many people with ostomies, like many normally-plumbed people, will want a remedy for diarrhea; those with colostomies may wish to pack a mild laxative. If you're heading for a hot, humid climate, you may want prescriptions for a fungicide to deal with any fungus problems around the stoma; the doctor or ET nurse can give you instructions for using it. Foresighted travelers who have ileostomies and are going to areas where tourist diarrhea is common pack some potassium chloride powder for electrolyte replacement drinks.

For any extensive trip, have prescriptions filled before you go and carry them in the original labeled container, especially if you will be going through customs. Some states and foreign countries do not honor prescriptions from your home state. Make a note of the generic name of each medicine (the drug's name without a registered trademark; *triamcinoline acetonide*, for instance, is the generic name for Kenalog[R]) in case of emergencies, and take along your doctor's name, address and phone number.

A "do not disturb" sign is helpful. Some people who irrigate their colostomies swear by a package of clip-on metal shower curtain hooks. These can be made into a chain of any length for hanging irrigation equipment from shower curtain rod, shower head or any sturdy (not a suction) hook.

If you're traveling in the U.S. or Canada, bring along the latest list of all UOA chapters (published as a separate section each year with the Winter issue of *Ostomy Quarterly*) in case you need help finding a pharmacy, physician, ET nurse or just someone to talk to. A directory of ET nurses is available from the International Association for Enterostomal Therapy (714-476-0268). The American or Canadian Cancer Society may also have information. If you're going abroad, check with the International Ostomy Association (c/o UOA) to locate groups in the countries you are visiting.

To sleep without worrying about accidents, pack a mattress cover of some type (it can be as simple as a large heavy plastic garbage bag to slip under the sheet). Water and cleansing agents in squeeze bottles make for pleasant, easy clean-ups along the way. Some travelers suggest packing your equipment at the time you are changing your pouch or irrigating, so you won't forget anything you need, whether your destination is Poughkeepsie or Rio de Janeiro.

Unless you're going only to places with a sure source of supply, take more supplies than you think you'll need. Be generous. Make a note of the name, size, order number and manufacturer of your basics and, just in case, take along the name and phone number of your pouch supplier. Many emergencies could be avoided by a quick call home and the speedy service of UPS or Federal Express.

Keep your supplies with you, or at least enough for 48 hours. A flight or carry-on bag or a briefcase can hold toilet necessities and a change of underwear as well as ostomy supplies. Never check your supplies through. Be sure they don't go astray by keeping them within arm's reach. (If you're flying, carry non-flammable solvent and adhesives to avoid having your trip interrupted by FAA inspectors.)

Comfortable wash-and-wear clothes are a boon for any traveler, including anyone with an ostomy. And while an extra change of clothing may make your suitcase a trifle heavier, it can increase your confidence.

A medical alert emblem or an emergency card belongs with you at all times, but especially when you travel. You can use a commercially-available warning or make your own with the vital information on it: what kind of an ostomy you have, any kind of medicine you are taking, and any special precautions (no enemas or rectal temperatures, for instance). Include a warning: "Do not remove ostomy pouch without doctor's orders."

Take it easy with what you eat and drink. Although digestive upsets are most often associated with foreign countries, they can follow a Chinese meal in San Francisco, a bowl of chili in Texas, or a double slab of pecan pie a la mode in Atlanta, particularly for the person with a rather new ostomy whose system is still used to simpler or blander fare.

Some people find they can eat anything and everything, and that's one of the pleasures of travel. Julia Schreier of Flushing, New York, has some wonderful gastronomic memories: "During the four strenuous weeks of go-go-going, not one bellyache, not one bout of indigestion or diarrhea did I experience. Indeed, I ate much more adventurously than my non-handicapped husband, drawing the line only at heavily spiced foods. Through two more subsequent trips, I have enjoyed broiled trout with platters of French fries in Geneva, spaghetti and meat sauce in Florence, cassata and gelati in Rome, Wiener schnitzel and pastry in Vienna, smoked salmon in Copenhagen, fish and chips in London, broiled scampi in a restaurant overlooking Michelangelo Square. . . ."

To avoid tourist diarrhea (a problem for many travelers who've never heard of an ostomy), follow the standard travel book instructions for the particular country—such as boiling water or avoiding certain fruits. If diarrhea strikes anyway, take your anti-diarrhea medication and stick to low-residue foods such as rice, soda crackers and bananas. Most important, drink *large* amounts of fluid to make up for the water and electrolyte loss: bouillon, tea with sugar, ginger ale. Drinking more fluids does not increase ostomy output for those with colostomies and ileostomies. Only urine output increases; the kidneys take care of balancing the body fluids.

Remember, too, those wise words of Satch Paige: "If your stomach disputes you, lie down and pacify it with cool thoughts."

For those with ileostomies and colostomies which discharge loose stools, dehydration occurs frequently and insidiously, especially during long car rides or summer traveling. Watch for weakness, thirst, decreasing urination. Better yet, prevent dehydration by drinking plenty of water and/or electrolyte-rich drinks. An immersion rod, a mug and a jug of water make fine hot drinks with tea bags, coffee and cocoa.

Expect the unexpected. That usually well-mannered colostomy or reasonably-docile ileostomy may act up a bit. The colostomy may require a drainable pouch for a day or two instead of a gauze square. Relax. Such troubles are usually temporary and, meanwhile, you're on your way!

For campers, motorists, airline and international travelers, some more-specific hints:

Campers rough it in varying degrees. Those who have self-contained recreational vehicles need make few adjustments for ostomies. Experienced campground campers suggest bringing plenty of toilet paper (as well as aluminum foil, newspaper or opaque plastic bags for disposing of used pouches). A waterproof rectangular plastic storage box (perhaps the kind meant to crisp celery and carrots in your refrigerator) works well both for storing supplies and for soaking reusable pouches. To avoid a chilly 3 a.m. trip to an outdoor privy, a number of campers suggest lining a large coffee can with a plastic bag, covering it with its own plastic lid and keeping it in your tent.

Victoria Campigotto from Ohio reports meeting a woman irrigating her colostomy in a camp bathhouse about five o'clock in the morning:

". . .There was a woman at the basin filling a colostomy irrigation bag and a one-half gallon thermos jug with warm water." After Victoria admitted to her new friend that 'I never had the nerve or the know-how to do it this way,' the woman showed her the equipment she had brought in her basket-type purse: regular paraphernalia plus water jug, a plastic funnel and a bent coat hanger which she bent into an over-the-door hook, with the hanger hook down, on which she hung her irrigating bag.

Ranging farther into the wilderness, people with ostomies continue to cope, using portable toilets with perhaps a tarp hitched between trees for privacy. Extremes in temperature cause some problems for some skin barriers, and may mean more frequent changes. A cooler works well for storage; a few drops of warm water will restore barriers that are too cold. Major changes in altitude may puff up plastic bottles storing cleaning supplies; squeezing out all the air before packing helps.

Veteran traveler Elnore Sturm, from St. Louis, tells of her experience on a 200-mile boat trip down the Colorado River with a group of 16 people. She switched to disposable equipment for her ileostomy during the trip and worried beforehand about maintaining her pouch. No bother! A portable chemical toilet placed behind a large boulder away from camp, together with a series of signals for when it was in use, provided relief for everyone, not just Elnore, during the night.

But: "The day was another story. We were instructed to drink plenty of water to remain hydrated as the temperature can get as high as 115 degrees and also were told that this would lead to 'pit' stops but would be no problem. We would have to ask to pull to the side when possible (on a small sand bar with some bushes or large rocks for privacy) and were to ask for the shovel, paper and matches!. . . I had to ask for a few extra stops, but no one except my husband really knew why! Colostomates would not be able to irrigate but would have to let nature take its course like the rest of the gang."

For traveling by car, seatbelts are safest when worn above or below the stoma; a long trip with a seatbelt rubbing the stoma directly may lead to irritation. But do wear them. As one doctor says, "I'd much rather fix an irritated stoma than massive internal injuries."

Glove compartments and trunks are usually too hot for supplies; a cooler or any place out of the sun works better. Since not all highway restrooms are well equipped, carry tissue, soap, hand towels, and wash cloths. An unscented spray deodorant or a lighted match, or a few drops of appliance deodorant can show thoughtfulness in the car or public restroom. Cloth pouch covers or even a large soft handkerchief placed between pouch and skin make for cooler, more comfortable traveling. So do cornstarch or talcum powder. And this is definitely the time to use that favorite cushion.

Air travel presents its own challenges. Those who wear metal faceplates may want to bring an extra faceplate and/or a doctor's statement in the language of countries to be visited to show security guards at the metal detector. You can request a private customs inspection if you wish.

Remember to empty pouches long enough before takeoff and landing to forestall ending up in a long line at the restroom. Emptying pouches relatively frequently while in flight also avoids problems, as does expelling air carefully from pouches and any tubes or plastic bottles of cement before takeoff.

Cross-country air travelers face the problem of jet lag, although not as severely as round-the-world travelers do. It's possible that a normally well-behaved colostomy may lag along with the rest of you. A day or so of adjustment to the new time zone should bring you back to a more normal schedule. Some people prefer to anticipate time zone changes, starting to change their irrigation schedule about a week beforehand if they irrigate. Some reports indicate that dehydration may contribute to jet lag. One jet plane crew member suggests drinking a glass of water every hour you're in a jet plane to counteract dehydration caused by cabin pressurization.

International boundaries prove no bar to those who have ostomies. Carol Norris, of Helsinki, Finland, tells of a year in Australia. After her surgery for a brief but brutal bout with ulcerative colitis and peritonitis, "ghoulish friends 'prepared' me never to be able to teach, dance, swim, or travel again. To prove them wrong, I did all those things, and added tenting. We camped from British Columbia to Newfoundland to Mexico and I toured Europe, sleeping with a girlfriend in a VW squareback. The Australia-Fiji year meant tenting for most of 40,000 miles, except for a few months in flats or cabin en route. . .I never sprang a leak, though I swam in the jellyfishy Coral Sea, slept on buses and slid down cliffs. Our wee tent became a snug home when things went 'bump,' 'screech,' 'thapthapthap' and 'heeheehahee' in the rainforests."

Besides writing novels and guides for the deaf and teaching English to Finnish students, Carol has added thousands more miles to her travel logs, including a summer from Scotland to Finland, quick visits to New York to see her agent and botanical expeditions in Death Valley.

Sandra Zarcades, of Del Mar, California, has an ileostomy. Faced with the chance to live in Greece for a year, she at first doubted her ability to cope: "My imagination conjured up a whole series of problems that could plague me: a terrible heat wave, intestinal flu, food blockage, and bouts of diarrhea." She reports a wonderfully stimulating year despite a few problems. She learned to sample new foods very cautiously. Because of hot climate, she always carried a canteen with her for shopping excursions and for walking tours, drinking from it frequently. She discovered new sources of potassium for herself in a country where frozen orange juice and bananas are rare: tomatoes in the summer and broccoli in the fall supplemented other foods.

International travelers have many resources they can call on. The International Association for Medical Assistance to Travelers (IAMAT), 417 Center Street, Lewiston, NY 14092, provides information on doctors, hospitals and such. The American Embassy, a Consulate, or a U.S. Military hospital in each country is another possible resource for U.S. citizens.

Get necessary shots well before bon voyage time, so any reactions will be well behind you when you leave.

What about water for irrigation or cleaning, as well as for drinking? A good rule of thumb is that anything that can go into your mouth can go into your stoma, but even clean water may contain bacteria that are unfamiliar to our systems. When there is any doubt, boil water (unless you are at a high altitude). Or purify it by adding to 1 quart of water either (a) 1 or 2 tablets of Halizone, (b) 2% tincture of iodine (5 drops if water is clear, 10 drops if water is cloudy), or (c) 10 drops of chlorine bleach—mix and let stand 30 minutes. In an emergency, travelers have used bottled mineral water or even beer for irrigating and report they work fine. (Leave any carbonated drink out overnight to remove the carbonation bubbles.)

One point for international travelers over 65 from the U.S.: Social Security Medicare does not cover health care expenses outside the U.S. It might be well to take out private health insurance for the duration of the journey. Contact your medical insurance company or the Passport Office for further information.

On the lighter side, *The Town Karaya*, a Nevada ostomy newsletter, suggests using an extra ostomy pouch on self or mate as a money belt!

So, whatever your destination, plan ahead, use the resources available to you, meet each moment as it comes, and bring back a few hints of your own to share with others.

And—have a wonderful time!

CHAPTER 26 ❖ *Enterostomal*
Therapy: A New
Profession

When a surgeon rearranged her personal plumbing
many years ago, Norma Gill had no intention of
getting into the profession of enterostomal therapy.
For one thing, there was no such profession.

Norma Gill was one of the ostomy pioneers. As a young
housewife in Akron, Ohio, pregnant with her third child,
she learned that she would need an ileostomy for her
severe ulcerative colitis. She already had some unhappy
notions about ostomies since her grandmother (at 74) had
had a colostomy for cancer a few years before. It had
been impossible to find ostomy equipment, and Norma
remembered her aunts dealing with clumsy piles of
dressings that never quite hid the odor.

At the time of her own surgery in 1954, Norma was
bedridden for many miserable months. "It was then that
I made a vow to God that if I ever got out of that mess
I'd devote the rest of my life to rehabilitation of ostomates."

And that's exactly what Norma Gill has done. First she made a name for herself as an ostomy volunteer in Akron. Then her surgeon, Dr. Rupert Turnbull of the Cleveland Clinic, learned of her interest.

In 1958, he put her to work helping his patients at the Clinic, and gave her new specialty a name—enterostomal therapy (*entero*: intestine; *stoma*: opening). The term stuck, which is how ET nurses got their title. In spite of a thousand problems, the results were so successful that in 1961 Dr. Turnbull suggested they start a School of Enterostomal Therapy so other people with ostomies could learn how to help.

About the same time Norma Gill was learning her unexpected profession in Cleveland and starting to teach, other people with ostomies around the country were not only telling themselves that "something must be done," but finding ways to do it. Among them was Jean Alvers, a young housewife in San Francisco with some experience in business administration until her acute illness led to an ostomy.

Although her surgeons did a fine job, they didn't know how to tell her to care for her new stoma, so Jean in desperation experimented with plastic bags from a deli-catessen, some tape used on airplane wings and other oddments, until she'd invented an appliance that worked for her. Her doctors, amazed and impressed, started asking her to help other patients.

Meanwhile, in Boston, Edith Lenneberg took a different route after her ostomy. A music teacher with small children at home, she helped found the Boston Ostomy Association in 1952 and then, in 1957, became the editor of the first national journal for people with ostomies, *The Ileostomy Quarterly*. Along with news (including a profile of Norma Gill after her appointment as an enterostomal therapist), professional articles and tips, the *Quarterly* printed the names of new ostomy groups as soon as they were formed, thus helping people find each other. (Later, in 1967, Edith would be persuaded to open the Stoma Rehabilitation Clinic at New England Deaconess Hospital in Boston.)

Although they knew the mushrooming need, those ostomy pioneers didn't have it easy in those early days. Thanks to such medical breakthroughs as antibiotics and better blood transfusion techniques, more and more patients were surviving ostomy surgery. However, advice on how to live with such changes was almost non-existent. Appliances were cumbersome, inefficient, and hard to find.

Hospitals didn't always take kindly to these newly-minted experts whose main prerequisite for training was neither an MD nor an RN, but a stoma. Many doctors and nurses ignored them as mavericks. And most patients, however much they needed them, didn't know that enterostomal therapists existed.

In 1962, a scatter of mutual aid ostomy groups around the country banded together as the United Ostomy Association. In 1968, Norma Gill and the growing number of ETs who attended the UOA conference in Phoenix, Arizona, were persuaded by Dr. Turnbull that they needed a firmer and more formal way to keep in touch than chance meetings, long-distance phone calls, and postcards.

They formed the North American Association of Enterostomal Therapists, later renamed the International Association for Enterostomal Therapy (IAET). This organization would hold them together, allowing them to share information, set standards of practice and certify schools for ET training. With such a professional approach, they hoped the medical profession would come to recognize their value.

Much has changed since then, although the commitment to serve the person with an ostomy has not. Having a stoma is no longer necessary for ET training—but being a registered nurse is now a prerequisite. Except for a few long-time ETs, all the ostomy professionals now practicing are ET nurses. Most have passed a certification examination in the specialty, a test they must retake every few years; if they wish, they can write CETN, for *certified enterostomal therapy nurse,* after their names. (Depending on what the entrance requirements were when they entered ET training, some ET nurses are licensed vocational or practical nurses and others are RNs without bachelor's degrees; those admitted into the program in recent years must have a bachelor's degree as well.)

As those with ostomies discover, ET nurses fill an enormous gap. Most hospital staff nurses are lucky if they have had a two-hour lecture on ostomies during their training, and many have never seen a stoma. As for doctors, former UOA officer Mike Schreiber said: "If [the surgeon] took the time to instruct each of his ostomy patients about ostomy care in minute detail, I wonder how many surgeries he would have to forego and how many lives might be sacrificed because he didn't have sufficient time to do the important surgical tasks he had been trained to do."

ET nurses know that—important as attitudes are— proper information about stoma care can mean the difference between a dreary, bitter life as a self-styled handicapped recluse, and a good full life as a normal person, eager to enjoy the new life an ostomy has made possible. The person with an ostomy needs to know about skin care and skin problems, the best pouches for a given stoma, techniques for irrigating if a person with a colostomy chooses that option, and a host of other nitty-gritty matters. These technical aspects of ostomy care, as well as psychological aspects of coping, are the heart of the ET nurse's domain.

Before surgery, ET nurses find time to explain what is going to happen and why, and to reassure patients and their families that this surgery they may never have heard of before is not the end, but a new beginning. Alone or with the surgeon, they find and mark the best stoma site before surgery. After surgery, they help the patient determine the best ways to cope with the new stoma, choose equipment, learn how to manage, and return to former activities and jobs. Along with this technical and practical know-how, there's emotional support for the person adjusting to such changes, and a willingness to be called about minor as well as major problems.

Besides teaching and counseling patients, ET nurses also can and do teach doctors and nurses, giving in-service training programs and organizing regional workshops. In addition, some are active in research, and many work closely with local UOA chapters.

Bobbie Brewer, a former UOA president as well as an ET, sees the ET nurse as ". . .more than a pouch changer. Much more. She (or he) is a rehabilitation worker in the fullest sense of that word, helping the patient return to a full life."

In 1958, there was one ET. Now, IAET numbers about 2500 ET nurse members, and there are many more "stoma nurses" around the world. Despite this, geography still makes the services of an ET nurse a luxury in many parts of the country. Several years ago, for instance, at Coos Bay, Oregon, the nearest ET nurse was hundreds of miles away, so the local UOA group arranged for an all-too-brief visit from a California expert.

Even in urban areas, many hospitals still don't have an ET nurse on the staff. Some hospitals deny the need or say they can't afford one; others are actively recruiting an ET nurse but can't fill the opening.

Some ET nurses have been attracted to the field because of the experience of a close family member or a friend. Others are recruited by hospitals from the ranks of staff or are encouraged by the American or Canadian Cancer Societies or the local UOA group. Empathy for the person acquiring an ostomy is still an admission requirement for the ET nurse candidate, with or without a stoma. (Students who don't have ostomies may wear pouches full of water to see how it feels.)

Personal experience with ostomy surgery is still responsible for many recruits, including Melba Connors. She was already an RN when she opened her eyes after emergency surgery resulting from ulcerative colitis to find herself with an ostomy. She told about her experience in the *American Journal of Nursing*: "Depression settled like a fog, separating me from the figures who came in and out of the room."

People told her it would be easy because she was herself a nurse. "'I'm not a nurse,' I screamed within myself. 'I'm a human being who is scared to death. I'm afraid my husband won't love me, my teenage children will reject me, and I'll smell bad and offend my friends. Help me!'"

Although her internist assured her that she could have a normal life, she did not believe him: "'Your idea of a normal life is different than mine,' I thought. 'I'll never wear tight clothes again. I'll have a restricted diet. How will I manage the care? Everyone who comes in takes care of it differently. . .!'"

As the hospital days dragged on and Melba encountered discomforts and complications—severe pain in the perineal wound, noise, non-stop gas, raw skin, a leaking appliance, and a roommate who called her "Stinky"—she plummeted deeper into depression, crying at night when she thought no one would hear.

Then, "One day the student nurse who was caring for me said casually, 'You know, my roommate has an ileostomy. Would you like to talk to her?' A student nurse with an ileostomy! 'Yes, of course, I'd like to see her.'

"Just after visiting hours, a darling young girl in a very tight, form-fitting dress walked in. 'Hi,' she said. 'I'm Sandy. My roommate said you would like to talk to me.' I was astounded. This vivacious, slim girl could not have an ileostomy! 'Sorry I'm late. I was just starved, so I stopped to pick up a pizza before I came!' A pizza! I thought of the horrible, bland diet I was eating and suspected she did not have a stoma at all."

She did, though, and her help in selecting a pouch as well as in showing what a person with an ileostomy could do proved the turning point for Melba: "With this appliance, I no longer had sore skin or accidents, and the odor was controlled. By now I could see quite a bit of blue sky."

An article in a nursing journal led Melba to her specialty, for she remembered those first frustrations—and what a blessing a little help was. After working with the Visiting Nurse Program in San Diego, she became director of an ET training program.

Bonnie Bolinger, RN, ET, who became a president of the ET organization, was drawn to ET training by her remembered anguish as a mother. When her daughter, Michelle, was six, she had to have a vesicostomy (a hard-to-manage type of urinary diversion). "The statement that registered most in my mind was, 'She will be the first child with the surgery in Dayton, Ohio!' Reassurance out the window—isolation to take its place.

"Isolation and lack of knowledge by the health care team left me wondering. Where was I to go for help? Who would understand my six-year-old's needs? Her goal was to enter first grade. The school didn't want her. The surgeon ordered equipment that would not fit an adult, much less a child.

"Anger, anger, anger at all concerned. Her vesicostomy looked crude, her abdomen appeared to have second degree burns, she hurt, I hurt, her father retreated, her brothers didn't understand all the tension and tears. I called my sister, an RN, and pleaded for her to take my first-born and relieve me of my anguish. My sister proceeded to wrap Michelle in a blanket and storm every doctor's office that had been involved with the case, demanding action.

"She got action! Three doctors called within two hours. Equipment was ordered and Mr. Botvin from Torbot Company taught me to care for Michelle over the phone. He conveyed knowledge, reassurance, and a hot-line number for follow-up care."

ET training came later when Michelle was 12 and the other children had reached school age. Though Bonnie wasn't sure she could handle the courses, she went to school to become a licensed vocational nurse. ET school came later, as did becoming an RN. Bonnie, like her daughter, was also a first—the first ET in Dayton, Ohio.

Gerry Cameron, RN, ET, doesn't have a stoma. However, when she began a hospital Patient Education Department, she was concerned about the lack of information for people who'd had ostomies. At a regional UOA meeting, she heard for the first time about the nursing specialty of enterostomal therapy.

For three months she pondered how she could manage the training, and then talked it over with her husband. He said she should apply in spite of many obstacles. These seemed to disappear like magic. Her best friend's folks lived in the city where the program was located; she could stay with them. The American Cancer Society provided the money. Her husband's cousin came to look after the family for the six weeks she'd be away, and her husband drove with her to the ET school, flying home and leaving her the car.

Gerry found the training very interesting. Since completing it, ". . .it has been my pleasure to work with many people with ostomies. Each one is a special person to me, and I continue to find my work a very rewarding experience."

Eunice Gaskell, RN, ET, was head nurse on a surgical floor of a California hospital. "I realized ostomy patients seemed frustrated, even with the teaching after surgery, so I told them to call me after they were home and had a problem. The phone calls began. So did the idea of further education and selling a program to the hospital and physicians. One of the satisfactions, since I've had my ET training, is being able to work with the patients and their families in the hospital and after discharge for continuity of care."

How does one become an ET nurse? Admission requirements at the few approved enterostomal therapy training schools are high: Currently, one must be an experienced registered nurse with a Bachelor's Degree, either in nursing or another field. (Requirements may change at any time, however.) The programs offer several weeks of "didactic" (instruction) along with variable amounts of clinical practice (in which the student puts new skills to work). A list of schools and entrance requirements is available from the International Association for Enterostomal Therapy, 27241 La Paz Road, Suite 121, Laguna Nigel, CA 92656; telephone (714) 476-0268.

What do ET students learn? Working with many specialists—including colorectal and urinary tract surgeons, dermatologists, dietitians, social workers, psychiatrists and ET nurses—students learn the anatomy and physiology of the many different kinds of ostomies. They observe surgery; learn to care for patients from before surgery through the hospital experience, discharge and beyond; teach patients, other health professionals and the general public; and attend meetings of local UOA chapters. Lectures alternate with observation and clinical practice. Supervision is close. It is almost an apprenticeship program, since most schools limit enrollment to a few students at a time.

The horizons of practice for ET nurses keep expanding. Now many ET nurses work not only with people who have ostomies, but also with patients who have draining wounds, diabetic or pressure ulcers ("bedsores"), incontinence, or impotence. The training reflects this broadening scope, although many ET nurses would like to see a longer "clinical internship" program so that students would learn more about these newer areas.

Many scholarships for ET training are available from ostomy supply manufacturers, the American Red Cross, and other sources. (UOA, for instance, offers the Archie Vinitsky Scholarship for ET Nursing Education.) Scholarship information is available from IAET.

After passing the certification exam, the new ET nurse returns home to a waiting job: working in a hospital, for several hospitals, with home care groups like Visiting Nurse Association, or in a stoma rehabilitation clinic. Some ET nurses are employed by ostomy supply manufacturers and private practice is another option. The expanded scope of practice has opened up other employment choices, such as wound or incontinence care. ET nurses may be paid a salary (usually higher than that of a staff nurse), earn a commission (for some ET nurses employed by industry), or may bill patients for services rendered. Some insurance plans cover enterostomal therapy; some do not. After joining IAET, the ET nurse has further resources, including refresher courses, annual conferences and the professional journal, *The Journal of ET Nursing*. Regional IAET divisions offer more support and activities.

Although the outlook for the rehabilitation of people with ostomies in the United States, Canada, and Western Europe has improved dramatically in the last several years, other countries are not as fortunate. Canada has its own Canadian Association for Enterostomal Therapy, and the number of trained stoma therapists is increasing in Western Europe and Australia. The rest of the world still has only a handful, however, along with some special problems. In a developing country, for instance, where a multi-generational family of eight or more may share one room, privacy is impossible. Sanitary facilities and ostomy supplies my be non-existent. Attitudes and cultural norms can also create problems. Prilli Stevens, RN, ET from Capetown, South Africa, reports that she's called "Bad Lady" by witch doctors who harass her.

In many countries, importing ostomy supplies is a problem because of prohibitive duties, bureaucratic hassles, and high taxes. Together with the International Ostomy Association, the World Council of Enterostomal Therapists is fighting such problems.

Trained UOA visitors and ET nurses complement each other. Several years ago, visitors from the local ostomy group—if one existed—were the only resource to help patients, so visitors gave the best answers they could to questions about appliance choice, skin care, and other matters. Margot Julian, RN, ET (who has an ileostomy herself and who has worked actively in UOA at both local and national levels) explains that the ET nurse ". . .is a trained specialist. . .whose profession is planning the rehabilitation of those who have had surgical diversion of the bowel or bladder. This involves counseling on the psychosocial aspects as well as the selection of prosthetic devices and instructions on their use. . . .

"The certified visitor is an ostomate who has been carefully selected and trained to 'help establish the patient's graceful acceptance of the stoma and speed his return to normal living.' Visitors should not give medical advice, provide nursing care, nor attempt to practice enterostomal therapy. Visitors can give something that can never be provided by a non-ostomate: living proof that there *is* life after surgery. . . .

"Through the years, in recognition of the fact that behind every stoma is a whole patient with other nursing needs, and for legal reasons, enterostomal therapy has evolved into a nursing specialty. The emergence of the enterostomal therapist released the ostomy visitor from the responsibility of providing advice on stoma management. This is an increasingly complex task as the technology improves its response to needs of ostomates largely as expressed through the UOA. At the same time, the trend toward non-ostomate RN-ETs makes it imperative that good visitors be available to do what they do best, to provide moral support on a one-to-one basis from someone who has 'been there.' "

The hours are long and the work is hard, but most ET nurses find great satisfaction in their jobs. Most are enthusiastic about the degree of autonomy they have, the prestige they enjoy, and the fact that they make an enormous difference in their patients' lives.

All too often, in addition to helping the person with a new ostomy, they must still rescue those who had their ostomy surgery a long time ago but who've had inadequate or no advice on how to manage. Melba Connors comments on some of the repair work an ET nurse runs into:

"I have visited people who had bought appliances over the counter in a surgical supply house. Leaking and odor were borne with stiff upper lips. They have never complained about their horrendous skin irritations. . .because they thought that everyone that had this surgery had the same problems."

Melba also tells a harrowing story about a woman who'd had a colostomy for twenty years. After surgery, she was taught to irrigate with a standard enema set-up and for 20 years had been confined to her home, using 10 quarts (liters) of water and spending six hours a day in the bathroom, lying over the toilet. "Fortunately, in one lesson, I was able to modify her equipment. . .provide her with an irrigating sleeve and the correct method of irrigation. . . .By the end of the week she had control and she was able to throw away her pouch forever. With tears in her eyes she thanked me for rescuing her from bondage. The tears in my eyes, though, were for the never-to-be-recovered 20 years that she had lost."

CHAPTER 27 ❄ *The Phoenix:*
UOA and Its Ancestors

How beauteous mankind is! O brave new world.
That has such people in it!
Shakespeare, *The Tempest*

No bells rang, no trumpets blared that February in 1949 when a handful of people with ostomies met in a hospital room near Philadelphia. They had no inkling that this would be the beginning of a movement which would sweep the United States, Canada and, eventually, the world.

They weren't concerned with triumphs of the future, but with solving immediate problems. "Successful" ostomy surgery had left them with intolerable problems: skin breakdown, primitive pouches and odor, among others. Worse still was the sense of isolation, of being different from everyone else. The name of the hospital—Valley Forge—seemed singularly appropriate. Like General Washington and his troops almost two centuries before, these people were facing a Valley Forge of illness, desolation, and near-despair.

Now they had found each other. Sharing experiences

and problems, they found solutions sometimes, moral support always.

That was the beginning. The late Ira Karon, a past president of the United Ostomy Association, wrote about the next steps: "...In February of 1950 the second group was formed in Los Angeles, and in 1951 QT New York came into being. These groups were formed, each without knowledge of the other and each was begun at the suggestion of a surgeon."

In the case of QT New York, the surgeon was Albert S. Lyons (who worked closely with UOA from that point on). Aware that his ileostomy patients were surviving surgery—but barely surviving the aftermath—he and hospital social worker Miss Lucy Neary set up a meeting of women with ileostomies from Ward T of Mount Sinai Hospital, New York City. At the third get-together, in the social work office at Mount Sinai, 15 people showed up, including men with ileostomies from Ward Q. Thus began QT New York.

Dr. George Schreiber joined QT in its first months. (Both he and Dr. Lyons faced the scoffs of other doctors who didn't like the idea of mutual-help groups for patients.) Within a few months, members were visiting new ileostomy patients in the hospital. A joint venture of QT New York and QT Boston, *QT Bulletin*, the first ostomy newsletter in the country, appeared early in 1952. That same year, Dr. Lyons and Dr. Schreiber opened the first stoma clinic in the nation, and Dr. Lyons wrote a letter, published in the *Journal of the American Medical Association*, about the success of this group approach.

New groups were springing up across the country: Boston, San Francisco, St. Paul, Minnesota, and elsewhere. In May, 1956, the first country-wide conference met in New York, with representatives from ten groups. Despite a push for unification, many representatives were reluctant to gather ileostomy and colostomy groups under a single banner. Participants relished their autonomy, but decided to keep in touch by publishing two national journals, one for people with colostomies and one for those with ileostomies. *The Ileostomy Quarterly*, edited by Edith Lenneberg of QT Boston, thrived (except financially); later it would become the *Ostomy Quarterly*. (The *Quarterly* was exchanged in bulk across the Atlantic for copies of the publication of the Ileostomy Association of Great Britain, an organization formed in 1956; not only in the U.S. was the ostomy mutual-help movement gathering steam.)

The time was not yet ripe for unification in 1956. There were too many worries about whether people with ileostomies and colostomies could really help each other, too many fears about losing local independence and control. (People with urinary ostomies weren't being considered at all yet.)

But the dream of unification did not die. Sam Dubin, a small, quiet, and gentle man who had suffered from ulcerative colitis for years before his ileostomy in 1952, became standard bearer for the dream: a national organization to weld local ostomy groups into a powerful force for everyone with an ostomy. He infected others with his commitment to a united association for mutual aid, moral support, education and communication.

A second national meeting, late in 1960, brought together over 400 members in New York. Don Binder, who would later become Executive Director of UOA, drove all night from Cincinnati to attend: "We talked at the meeting about organizing a national association, but nothing was resolved. When time ran out, some of us gathered that evening. . .to continue discussion. . . A steering committee was established, and they met the following year in Detroit to make further plans."

Archie Vinitsky, President of the St. Paul's Colostomy and Ileostomy Rehabilitation Guild, Inc., of Minnesota, led the Detroit meeting. Participants struggled to define purposes for a national organization—which local groups would accept. They decided that a national organization, without interfering with the aims and autonomy of the local chapters, "could act as a clearinghouse of ideas and information for all clubs, could standardize a visiting program for greater helpfulness, could better reach the medical and lay public, could encourage research with greater financial resources, could stop wasteful duplication of effort, and could more effectively aid in the rehabilitation of people with ostomies." (Chairman Vinitsky would later serve as President of UOA; in the 1970s, he would guide the fledgling International Ostomy Association as its first President.)

Next stop was Cleveland, Ohio, for the Constitution Convention in 1962. Norma Gill, working full time at the Cleveland Clinic as the first stoma therapist, took on the task of organizing the Convention: "The first meeting in Cleveland was decided on at the last minute in Detroit when we all realized it was either now or never in forming a national association. Time doesn't permit [even mentioning] all our problems at that first convention, since there were no guidelines, no money and only our new Cleveland group."

Nevertheless, 115 representatives and six ostomy supply exhibitors attended the Convention on September 22, 1962. The name United Ostomy Association—Don Binder's suggestion—was accepted; national officers were elected. There was sadness too: In August, one month before his dream was to become a reality, Sam Dubin died of heart failure. In his memory, UOA would later name its highest honor the Sam Dubin Achievement Award.

The growing pains continued. Don Binder resumes the story: "My feeling when we left Cleveland was very doubtful that we would survive the first year. But 28 chapters affiliated and when we gathered the following

September in Los Angeles for the 1st Annual Convention we had survived and had confidence that the Association would grow."

During this 1st UOA Annual Convention, the Board of Directors voted $2500 for publication of a magazine devoted to ostomy problems. As Virginia Pearce Geiger (editor of the *Ostomy Quarterly* from its first issue, December 1963, until she resigned in 1978) recalls: "All jobs had to be done on a voluntary basis.

"Separated by over 2000 miles and working in their spare time, the editor and business manager had to establish format, obtain copy and advertising, do the artwork, layout, printing and distribution of the magazine, plus solving a myriad of problems. However, without sufficient funds to finance the enterprise, the decision was made to proceed, because all concerned felt that the great need for such a publication far outweighed the obstacles to be overcome."

Those who were in at the beginning still catch their breath when they realize how far UOA has come. Dave Slutzky, for instance, one of the original group which met near Philadelphia in 1949, attended the 10th Annual Conference in San Francisco in 1972, where almost 1000 conferees gathered. He and the others listed as participants in the first national conference in 1956—some of whom continue to serve, year after year, as the sturdy backbone of UOA—still find it hard to believe that the organization now numbers tens of thousands of members, in hundreds of chapters spanning the United States and Canada.

No matter how large it becomes, however, UOA cannot forget that it is a collection of local chapters and satellite groups. These are self-supporting units with their own membership and officers. Monthly meetings, open to everyone, usually include a talk or panel discussion by doctors, nurses, and/or people with ostomies. There are displays of ostomy products, and plenty of discussion afterwards around the coffee pot, as everyone gets acquainted. Chapters publish their own newsletters, and encourage publicity in newspapers, radio, and television. With the help of medical advisors and ET nurses, many chapters present in-service programs in hospitals.

Local chapters, often with the help of the local Cancer Society unit, train members to visit patients in hospitals and homes before and after ostomy surgery. Thousands upon thousands of people remember that first breath of hope that blew in with a UOA visitor—smiling proof that a normal life was within reach after ostomy surgery. With the development of ET nurses well versed in technical know-how, UOA's Visitor Training Programs have changed. There's more concern about psychological support, less with "which bag is best."

As strength and health return, many people with new ostomies bring their questions and doubts to the local chapter meeting. And, as they become relative old-timers, many stay, passing on their experience and support to help newer members.

The UOA is sectioned geographically into regions. A regional coordinator supervises other volunteers, who work directly with established chapters and develop new groups where they are needed. Each region holds annual or biannual conferences (called a conference rather than a convention to emphasize the educational programs and the seriousness of intent).

Regional programs dovetail snugly with the national program, which has headquarters in Southern California. Volunteer national officers and a Board of Directors, all elected at the annual conference, decide on policy and new directions for UOA.

A paid executive director and a small staff oversee various administrative activities. UOA publishes booklets and guides on ostomy care (as well as the *Ostomy Quarterly*), and provides charts, slides, and films. Among its activities, the national office guides national public relations, publicity, and fund-raising; keeps current membership lists; and handles correspondence. The office also supports the efforts of the national committees planning an annual Youth Rally and the annual UOA conference, which brings together those with ostomies, the medical professions, and often spouses and children. (The local chapters also get very involved in planning these two major events.) While it does not have its own funds for research, UOA cooperates with organizations which do.

UOA relies on a Medical Advisory Board, composed of doctors and ET nurses, for information and advice on medical issues. An Industry Advisory Board, with representatives from large and small manufacturers and suppliers, keeps UOA abreast of new developments in ostomy equipment.

At the Constitution Convention in 1962, the delegates reluctantly (even apologetically, recalls Don Binder), asked for annual dues of 50¢. Although the fee has gone up a bit since then, it's still low. Local chapters collect dues, then send on a portion to the national office. Large gifts and grants are rare. Volunteer effort is what makes UOA survive—and thrive.

Marilyn Mau, a former president of UOA, says that the recent years in UOA have seen "a change from the constantly increasing numbers of new chapters to a concentrated effort on supporting and strengthening the already existing ones. The number of members leveled off, and the aspect of membership retention became more important than ever. The UOA also began to expand its focus. Surgical alternatives to the standard ostomy surgery became available, and the need to ensure that the patient had a choice and was well-educated with respect to all the choices became apparent. 'Alternate Procedures' groups were embraced by UOA." (These groups offer information and support to people with ileoanal anastomosis with reservoir procedures, continent ostomies, and other alternative surgeries.)

UOA is reaching out to other groups with particular needs, as well. Children with ostomies (and their parents) can turn to special UOA groups. Teenagers can attend a rousing annual Youth Rally, which combines fun, new friendships and skills, information, and plenty of hugs and emotional support; IAET, the association of ET nurses, helps with the UOA-sponsored rallies.

Single adults can choose panel discussions and social events of their own at the annual conference. Older adults (over 62) may have special events at the conference. Homosexual and bisexual people with ostomies have the Gay and Lesbian Concerns Committee.

A continuing focus of the UOA is cooperation with other organizations and health care professionals to ensure that the person with an ostomy gets the best, most complete care possible. For instance, while ET nurses give instruction and physical care to the person with an ostomy, UOA contributes the "I've been there" moral support that *only* another person with an ostomy can provide. Close collaboration with the American and Canadian Cancer Societies and with such organizations as the Digestive Diseases National Coalition (DDNC) means that more patients are better served.

As the world shrinks, UOA strengthens its international ties as a supporter of the World Council of Enterostomal Therapy and as a member of the International Ostomy Association (IOA). In 1975, IOA became the umbrella organization for ostomy groups all over the world. In England, in Nigeria, in India, around the globe, people with ostomies are finding themselves no longer alone.

IOA has some special priorities, besides helping individuals and reaching the public with information about ostomies. Customs duties and import taxes, for example, remain hobgoblins, sometimes blocking the distribution of pouches and products across national borders.

The international cooperation works both ways. UOA, for instance, has been the lead organization in Project SHARE, which sends ostomy supplies to underdeveloped nations. Traveling in the other direction, information, inspiration, and good ideas from chapters around the world roll into the U.S. and Canada: revolutionary surgical techniques, useful equipment, new ways of meeting problems.

Why do people with ostomies even need such a group? Edith Lenneberg asked the question as part of a research project she conducted from 1958 to 1962: "Are they so immersed in self-pity that they need to withdraw and seek the company of commiserators; or does our society with its emphasis on 'normalcy' push them into a society-for-the-common-defense?" Edith concluded that ostomy and other mutual-help groups ". . .are the outgrowth of the increasing participation of the American public in matters of physical and emotional well-being. . .as a healthy effort at self-help towards the ultimate goal of. . .maximal self-dependence."

An ostomy group, thus, is a healthy step toward helping oneself—and then toward helping others. *Together*, people with ostomies have achieved what they could not have achieved alone. Without group pressure and in-genuity, many people would still be grappling with a smelly, one-size-fits-all pouch, constantly reddened weepy skin, odor, and other problems. Worst of all, they would be *alone* in the struggle, without support and practical advice.

Thanks to the efforts of thousands of people over many years, ostomy surgery, once considered "a fate worse than death," has become a chance for new life. Patients not only get well—they get "weller than well." They may expand the horizons of their lives: reaching out to others, accomplishing what might have daunted them before, using wisely the gifts of time and health that ostomy surgery has brought them.

To celebrate this rebirth "from the ashes of disease," UOA chose the phoenix as its symbol. Every five hundred years, this mythical, magical bird, knowing it is time to die, enters its nest of sweet-smelling myrrh, and rustles its glowing golden wings. The glow smolders into flame and the phoenix is consumed in a fiery holocaust. But as the glow fades, one spark rekindles, and then another— and from the ashes emerges the new phoenix: magnificent, towering, immortal.

Larry Litwack, the first president of UOA, wrote:. . ."The Phoenix represents a fiery symbol of the spirit and feeling underlying the growth of the Association. For the ostomate, what more appropriate choice could have been made? From the ashes of despair and disease, from the fear of disability and death, from the ebb tide of physical and emotional being to the full flood of life—of hope—of health. Reborn to a life of fulfillment—of dedication—of giving to others. Although not ourselves immortal as was the legendary bird, we gain perhaps true immortality by giving of ourselves to others, so that we live on forever in the hearts and minds of others."

Was it entirely a coincidence that the small town near Philadelphia where that first ostomy group gathered in 1949—was Phoenixville?

CHAPTER 28 ✣ *In the Family*

Caring is the greatest thing,
Caring matters most.
Freiderich Von Hugel

When Mother phoned that March dusk in 1976, her spirits matched the weather outside.

Dismal.

She tucked in an alarming snippet of news near the end of a sprawling and woeful conversation: ". . .just a little bit of blood in my bowel movement. Probably nothing to worry about."

But she was scared. And so was I, despite my casual, "Yeah, probably not serious. Do keep an eye out though, just in case it happens again. Okay?"

Our fears crouched behind a veil of mutual reassurance. Never in my memory had Mother so much as mentioned the bowel—her own or anyone else's.

And I? With two months to go before graduation from nursing school, I would have had to be a real dimwit not to have recognized the possible seriousness of such a complaint in a woman over 50 who'd never had even a whisper of trouble with her digestive tract.

A woman who happened to be very special to me.

Sure, it might be hemorrhoids. Maybe I was over-reacting.

Maybe. . .

A free-lance writer, Mother had little money and no doctor of her own. I confided my forebodings to a doctor friend who knew some of the community resources available. An appointment was arranged.

But Mother turned skittish. It took a few months and some canceled appointments before she finally had the physical exam. I fumed and fussed. Patient's rights or no, sometimes I was tempted to hogtie her, if necessary, to get her to the doctor.

We were both playing at make believe. To Mother, it was, as she would acknowledge later, a matter of "Until I see the doctor, there's nothing really wrong with me."

And I was striking my own bargain with Whomever had charge of these matters: If I just concentrated hard enough on the worst that could happen—why then, it wouldn't happen. Simple as that.

In late June Mother finally had her physical. She was jubilant over the results, and so was the doctor.

Until that sigmoidoscopy a few days later. I had driven her to the appointment and sat outside the office. When I saw the doctor's face as he barreled out of his office and sprinted up the stairs (to get another doctor to take a look), I *knew*.

When the biopsy report came back a few days later, I had to do something, take some kind of action. I knew next to nothing about ostomies. I'd been "exposed" to the subject, by way of a brief and boring film two years earlier, but that was it. I had never taken care of anyone with an ostomy, nor (to my knowledge) known anyone with this unfamiliar rearrangement of internal plumbing. All I had was a vague memory of some organization for people with ostomies.

A couple of phone calls later, I discovered that the local chapter of the United Ostomy Association, which met in San Francisco once every two months, was meeting that night. And what a meeting! It was the breath of hope I sought: There *was* life after an ostomy! *Good, full life.*

When Mother entered the hospital, my life took on the pace—if not the laughs—of a Keystone Cops comedy. The doctors first scheduled Mother's surgery for Thursday, the day I had to be in Sacramento taking the *surgery* test for my nursing State Boards (the two days of licensing examinations that one must pass to become a registered nurse). For assorted reasons, including my pleas, the surgeons postponed the operation until 7:00 a.m. Monday. I still remember very little about the Boards (but I did pass).

Sunday evening, a telegram arrived from my brother-in-law and his family in Indonesia: "Arriving San Francisco International 8:00 a.m. Monday."

I promptly burst into tears. "Tell me this isn't happening," I howled to Art, my husband. Later, I would be able to laugh. But not yet.

After a dawn visit to the hospital, staying until Mother's pre-operative medication relaxed her, I scrambled out to the airport to meet my exhausted in-laws, including two babies. I fear I was less than the perfect hostess.

Bless Dick and Judy, weary as they were, for being so understanding during their visit. And bless my friend Marcia, who showed up at the hospital to share the vigil outside the operating room. And Art and our children who, while facing their own feelings about Grandma's illness, helped so much.

In some ways, the pace of those few days cushioned the event for me. I had so many other things to worry about that I didn't have to face what was happening to Mother or how I was reacting to it.

Sometimes I retreated into my brand new "nurse" self when it became too painful to be a "daughter" self. The "nurse" self tried to encourage Mother to talk about what she was feeling—when the "daughter" self didn't necessarily want to hear. And occasionally, I fear, the plain old "me" self got lost in the shuffle.

But I did the "right" things, said the "right" words—and congratulated myself on how beautifully I was coping. I really was handling this *very* well.

Hah!

As my friend Carole says, "What 'I'm really handling this well' means is 'I haven't even begun to face this problem yet'!"

How right she is. My comeuppance came quickly. Three days later, a woman died on our ward. It was the first time I had ever been with a dying person—and she happened to be exactly the same age as my mother, and to have the same diagnosis. Woodenly, I carried out the tasks afterward.

When my work shift ended, I walked out to the parking lot. The tears began streaming.

For a week, I couldn't walk into the hospital to work without starting to cry. I wore a rut between the front door and the nearest bathroom, where I would sit and bawl.

But eventually I was all cried out.

One day, the food tasted like corrugated cardboard and paste. The next day, it was real food again, the chicken succulent, the salad crisp and delicious. San Francisco isn't exactly noted for its tree-lined streets, but what trees and blooms there were—I was *seeing*.

It was as if by confronting my worst fears (unwillingly, to be sure) I had begun to move through them and beyond them. Only then could I start concentrating on *today*, with its many joys and victories.

I kept asking myself why I hurt so much. After all, it was Mother who was miserable those first days after surgery, Mother who was having to learn all about living with an ostomy (although the ostomy itself was surprisingly little bother), Mother who was living with a scary diagnosis.

But we relatives and spouses and friends hurt too and

there doesn't seem to be any way to bypass that grieving. Instead, we struggle to find a path through it and beyond it. There are no "good" ways or "bad" ways: We are all different persons and our ways must be our own.

Why do we hurt? For many reasons.

Illness is itself a change and it brings about other changes. Relationships shift; that person we've always counted on—is now depending on us. We may feel left in the lurch, with crushing responsibilities and no one to share them. When someone close to us becomes seriously ill, we see our own vulnerability and mortality. That is frightening indeed. And we feel *with* the person who is ill, sharing the sorrow and the anger that this has happened.

As if all that weren't enough, we may feel anger at this person for being ill: for disrupting our lives, for worrying us, for draining our time, perhaps, or our energy and resources.

That anger may be quite normal, but it's pretty hard to accept in ourselves. After all, how can we be angry at someone for being sick? Enter the guilt.

I wish I could say I have it all figured out. I don't. All those nice pigeonholed "stages" of grieving that my nursing textbooks warned me about—were never that neat.

They still aren't.

Feelings—my feelings anyway—tend to be a hodge-podge of sadness and fear, with generous dollops of anger, resentment, and sometimes self-pity thrown in. Not to mention guilt, for all that anger, resentment, and self-pity!

Sometimes I get exasperated and sometimes I get plain furious: "Why does she have to question *everything?*" or "Why did this have to happen?"

But time and tears have helped.

Now, often, there's a real sharing, of thoughts, of feelings, of those wispy flights of fancy, of terrible jokes—and of a deep love. That edge of illness makes the good times far sweeter.

I'm proud of my mother, for what she's done, how she's coped, what she is.

She may be missing a section of her intestine.

But she's got *plenty* of guts.

ADDRESSES TO KNOW

American Cancer Society (ACS)
1599 Clifton Road, NE
Atlanta, GA 30329
(404) 320-3333
(local chapters in towns and cities)

Canadian Association for Enterostomal Therapy
621-740 Corydon Avenue
Winnepeg, Manitoba R31 0Y1
Canada

Canadian Cancer Society (CCS)
10 Alcorn Avenue, Suite 200
Toronto, Ontario M4Z 3B1
Canada
(416) 961-7223
(local chapters in towns and cities)

Cancer Information Service (CIS)
(a service of the National Cancer Institute)
1-800-4-CANCER

Crohn's and Colitis Foundation of America, Inc. (CCFA)
444 Park Avenue South, 11th Floor
New York, NY 10016-7374
1-800-343-3637
(formerly the National Foundation for Ileitis and Colitis, Inc.)

Consumer Information Center
Pueblo, Colorado 81009

Help for Incontinent People (HIP)
P.O. Box 544
Union, SC 29379

International Association for Enterostomal Therapy (IAET)
27241 La Paz Road, Suite 121
Laguna Nigel, CA 92656
(714) 476-0268

International Association for Medical Assistance to Travelers (IAMAT)
417 Center Street
Lewiston, NY 14092
(716) 754-4883

International Ostomy Association
(Check United Ostomy Association for current address)

National Coalition for Cancer Survivorship
1010 Wayne Avenue, 5th Floor
Silver Spring, MD 20910
(301) 585-2616

United Ostomy Association (Canadian Office)
5 Hamilton Avenue
Hamilton, Ontario L8V 2S3
(416) 389-8822

United Ostomy Association (U. S. Office)
36 Executive Park, Suite 120
Irvine, CA 92714-6744
1-800-826-0826

GLOSSARY

ABDOMINOPERINEAL RESECTION (A-P Resection). Surgical procedure in which all or part of the colon and the entire rectum and anus are removed. The end of the remaining intestine is then brought through the abdominal wall as a permanent ostomy. If part of the colon is removed, this is a colostomy; if all of the colon is removed, the resulting ostomy is an ileostomy. The procedure is named after the two incisions necessary: one through the abdomen and the other through the perineum (the area between the genitals and the anus).

ANASTOMOSIS. Connection of two body parts by joining them surgically (e.g., removing a segment of colon and anastomosing the two remaining ends).

ANTI-REFLUX VALVE. With a urostomy, a way to keep urine from backing up into the kidneys. In a continent urostomy, a one-way valve is constructed at the inlet of reservoir to do this. Many external urostomy pouches incorporate an anti-reflux system to draw and store urine away from the stoma.

APPLIANCE. See POUCH

ASCENDING COLOSTOMY. See COLOSTOMY.

BARIUM ENEMA. Special x-ray examination of the lower digestive tract. Thick liquid substance, inserted through anus or colostomy stoma, fills colon and makes it show up clearly on x-ray films taken during procedure. Similar procedure, done through ileostomy stoma, is called small bowel barium enema.

BIOPSY. Removing a piece of tissue from a living body and examining it under a microscope to diagnose disease.

BLOCKAGE. See OBSTRUCTION.

BOWEL PREP. The use of diet, laxatives and/or enemas to prepare the digestive tract before a test or surgery involving the bowel. Removing any stool makes the intestine easier to see (for a test), or much cleaner (for surgery). Antibiotic pills are a part of the bowel prep before surgery.

BRICKER LOOP. See ILEAL CONDUIT.

BROOKE ILEOSTOMY. See ILEOSTOMY, CONVEN-TIONAL.

CARCINOGENIC EMBRYONIC ANTIGEN (CEA). Blood test for a specific protein, done periodically for people treated for colorectal cancer. If the blood level of CEA is higher than normal at the beginning of treatment, it can be checked later to help tell how effective treatment is. Can also be used to alert doctor to a possible return of the disease.

CECOSTOMY. Insertion of a tube through the skin into the cecum (cul-de-sac at beginning of large intestine) to remove gas or feces. Temporary procedure, some-times (but rarely) done to protect new surgical site in the colon while it heals.

COLECTOMY. Removal of colon (large intestine), either in part (partial colectomy) or all of it (total colectomy).

COLONIC CONDUIT. One type of operation to divert

urine away from the bladder. Short section of colon is cut away from the rest of the intestine, along with its blood and nerve supply. Section is closed at one end, ureters are attached to it, and open end is brought through abdominal wall to form stoma. Section thus becomes conduit (passageway) for urine to exit the body. Remaining ends of intestine are reconnected and resume function of moving feces out of body.

COLONOSCOPY. Insertion of long, flexible, lighted tube through anus (or through stoma) into colon to see if there is disease visible anywhere in the large intestine. Biopsy specimens can be obtained or polyps can be removed through the colonoscope.

COLOPROCTECTOMY (Proctocolectomy). Removal of all or part of the colon and all of the rectum.

COLORECTAL CANCER. Cancer of colon or rectum. Common cancer in people over 45. Most common reason for permanent colostomy.

COLOSTOMY. Surgical construction of new opening on abdomen for large intestine. This can be permanent (if the rectum and anus are removed) or temporary. (Also see TEMPORARY OSTOMY.) Colostomies are named by their location in the colon:

Ascending colostomy. Opening in ascending colon. Rare, temporary ostomy. Pouch needed at all times.

Transverse colostomy. Opening in transverse colon. Stoma located on upper abdomen usually at or above the waistline. Temporary procedure. Pouch worn at all times.

Descending colostomy. Opening in descending colon. May be permanent (if sigmoid colon, rectum and anus are removed also) or temporary. Stoma usually on left side of abdomen, below waistline. Occasionally managed with irrigation, but usually with pouch worn at all times.

Sigmoid colostomy. Opening in sigmoid colon. Most common permanent colostomy, but can be temporary if rectum and anus are left. Stoma usually on lower left abdomen below waistline. Managed with irrigation or pouch.

COMPUTED TOMOGRAPHY (CT scan). Technique for making cross-sectional images of internal body parts. An x-ray beam from a computerized scanner is passed through the body at different angles; the images are then assembled by computer. The patient lies on a table while the scanner rotates around the table. Sometimes medicine is injected into the vein to show body parts more clearly.

CONE. Part of colostomy irrigation set. Soft, plastic cone-shaped piece at end of tubing, fits snugly against stoma to keep irrigation fluid in the colostomy.

CONTINENT ILEOSTOMY (Continent intestinal reservoir, CIR, Kock pouch). Surgical variation on ileostomy. Surgeon loops part of the ileum back on itself and, by cutting loop open, refolding and stitching it, constructs a reservoir inside abdomen; a small tube made of ileum leads from reservoir through abdominal wall to form small stoma, flat on the skin. One-way valve at exit of reservoir keeps feces in the reservoir except when a catheter (plastic or rubber tube) is inserted a few times each day to drain feces; gauze pad or bandaid covers the stoma at other times. Can be done as curative surgery for ulcerative colitis or familial polypsis or as a conversion procedure for the person with a conventional ileostomy.

CONTINENT UROSTOMY (Urinary Kock pouch or Indiana pouch). A kind of urinary diversion. Internal reservoir constructed as in continent ileostomy, but with ureters attached. Additional valve at junction of ureters and reservoir to prevent urine from backing up into the kidneys (anti-reflux valve). Urine is drained from the reservoir a few times a day with a catheter inserted through the stoma; a gauze pad or bandaid is worn the rest of the time. Kock pouch is made from last section of ileum; Indiana pouch uses small piece of ileum and segment at beginning of large intestine.

CONVEXITY. A pouching technique for a stoma that does not protrude well. A firm molded faceplate curves against the body around the stoma, making a tighter pouch-skin seal and pushing the stoma out somewhat.

CROHN'S DISEASE (Ileitis, regional enteritis, granulomatous disease of bowel, Crohn's colitis). One of the inflammatory bowel diseases. Typically affects entire thickness of loop of bowel. Most often found in last part of ileum (ileitis), but can be found anywhere in the digestive tract; abdominal pain and diarrhea are most common symptoms. Can cause symptoms elsewhere in the body. Sometimes treated with an ileostomy, but it can recur after surgery. Disease is chronic and the cause is unknown. Crohn's colitis is Crohn's disease involving colon.

CYSTECTOMY. Removal of the bladder, either part (partial cystectomy) or all of it (total cystectomy).

CYSTOSCOPY. Insertion of a small rigid or flexible tube through the urethra into the bladder to see if there is any disease visible. Biopsy specimens can be taken through the cystoscope.

DIGESTIVE TRACT (Gastrointestinal tract, GI tract, alimentary canal). The hollow tube which goes from the mouth to the anus. Through it, food is taken into the body and broken down for use, and then the waste products are eliminated. Consists of the mouth, esophagus, stomach, small intestine, colon, rectum, and anus.

Small intestine. Approximately 20-22 feet (6.5-7 m) of coiled bowel where most digestion takes place, consisting of *duodenum*, 10-12 inches (25-30 cm) long, beginning at outlet of stomach; *jejunum*, about 8 feet (2.5 m) long; *ileum*, about 12 feet (3.5 m) connecting to large intestine at pouch called *cecum.*

Large intestine. Approximately six feet (2 m) of large bowel (wider in diameter than small intestine) where some absorption of water and salts takes place and the waste is stored for elimination. Begins at cecum in right lower abdomen, ascending to right rib area (*ascending colon*), crossing to left rib area (*transverse colon*), descending along left side (*descending colon*), slanting across left groin to mid-pelvis (*sigmoid colon*), descending along spine (*rectum*) to outlet (*anus*).

DOUBLE-BARREL OSTOMY. Type of ostomy (usually temporary) in which the intestine is severed, and both severed ends are brought through abdominal wall to form separate stomas. (Segment of intestine may be removed.) Stomas may be close to each other or not.

One stoma, still connected to the food-digesting part of the intestinal tract, discharges feces; the other, the mucous fistula, no longer connected to the functioning digestive tract, may discharge a small amount of mucus or may discharge nothing.

ELECTROLYTE.   Chemical compounds (such as salt) which dissolve in body fluids to form particles with an electric charge. They are needed in small amounts and in the right balance to maintain normal body functioning. If electrolytes are out of balance, a person may become weak and ill, and may need electrolyte supplementation by mouth or through a vein.

ENCRUSTATION.   Deposits of gritty urine crystals on urostomy stoma or skin around stoma. Prevented by drinking lots of fluids, keeping urine acidic and protecting all skin around stoma with correctly-fitted pouch. Treatment is half-strength vinegar soaks (one part water to one part vinegar), either with compresses applied directly to area or solution inserted into ostomy pouch.

ENDOSCOPY.   Examination of hollow organ in body by means of a lighted tube. Esophagus, stomach and part of the small intestine can be visualized with endoscope inserted through the mouth. Colonoscopes, sigmoidoscopes, and cystoscopes are some other types of endoscopes.

END OSTOMY.   An ostomy with a stoma with a single opening. The digestive tract or urinary tract is severed and the functional end is brought through the abdominal wall as a stoma (as opposed to a loop ostomy).

ENTEROSTOMAL THERAPY NURSE (ET nurse).   Health professional with special training in ostomy care and related fields. Currently, people accepted into an ET training program must be RNs with a Bachelor's degree in nursing or other field; they complete a six-to-eight week (or longer) course in an accredited enterostomal therapy program and pass a certification examination. Originally, ETs did not need to be nurses, but did have to have an ostomy. An ostomy is no longer required, and the educational requirements for admission to an ET program are being changed frequently; depending on when the person entered ET training, there is a wide variation in the amount of nursing background. ET nurses have expanded their practice to include such areas as draining wounds, pressure sores, and incontinence. Nurses who have passed the certification examination may call themselves certified enterostomal therapy nurses (CETNs).

ENTEROSTOMY. Any ostomy in the digestive tract.

EXCORIATION. For people with ostomies, it refers to red, raw, sore skin around stoma, often from enzymes in loose feces.

EXCRETORY UROGRAPHY. See INTRAVENOUS PYELOGRAM.

FAMILIAL POLYPOSIS (Familial polyposis coli, familial adenomatous polyposis, hereditary multiple polyps). Disease passed down in families; the large intestine contains huge numbers of polyps which become cancerous over time. To prevent cancer, the colon is removed; the rectum (all or the surface layer) is usually removed. An ileostomy (either conventional or continent), ileorectal anastomosis (ileum to rectum) or an ileoanal reservoir are options.

FECES (Stool, bowel movement). Bodily wastes which are discharged through anus or through colostomy and ileostomy stomas.

FISTULA. An abnormal tract (passage) between a body organ and the skin or between two body organs. These are a frequent complication of Crohn's disease. (See also MUCOUS FISTULA, surgically-created planned fistula.)

FLUSH STOMA. Stoma flat with skin level. Desirable with continent ostomy; may be difficult to manage with conventional ileostomies and some colostomies.

FOLLICULITIS. Inflammation of the hair follicles. Can be caused around stoma by ripping body hair off when pouches are removed or by shaving closely with safety razor.

GARDNER'S SYNDROME. A disease passed down in families; marked by multiple polyps in the large intestine and other abnormalities. Polyps have high potential for becoming cancerous. Colon and rectum are often removed to prevent colorectal cancer. Part of familial adenomatous polyposis syndrome.

GRANULOMATOUS DISEASE OF THE BOWEL. See CROHN'S DISEASE.

HARTMANN'S POUCH. A surgical option for a temporary ileostomy or colostomy. The intestine is severed, and the functional end is brought through the abdominal wall as a stoma which discharges stool. The remaining end (which leads to the anus) can be stitched or stapled shut and left in the abdomen as a blind-end Hartmann's pouch. The surgical procedure is called *Hartmann's procedure.*

HERNIA (Parastomal hernia, peristomal hernia). Protrusion of intestine through abdominal muscles around stoma. Seen as a bulge under the skin around stoma. May be supported with wide belt or binder; sometimes needs surgical correction.

HYPERPLASIA (Epidermal hyperplasia). "Warty" looking gray thickening of skin that can occur around urostomy stoma. Caused by alkaline urine, incorrectly-fitted skin barrier/pouch, and/or lack of night drainage system.

ILEAL CONDUIT (Bricker loop, ileal loop). Urinary diversion operation which allows urine to pass from kidneys via ureters through passageway made of short segment of small intestine to outside of body. Similar to colonic conduit except that ileum is used instead of colon. Stoma usually on lower right abdomen. Commonest permanent urinary diversion.

ILEITIS. See CROHN'S DISEASE.

ILEOANAL PULL-THROUGH PROCEDURE. Surgical procedure in which the colon and the surface layer of the rectum are removed and the ileum is pulled through the rectal "sleeve" and attached to the anus. The last part of the ileum is usually made into a reservoir; without a reservoir, the frequency and looseness of stool cause major management problems for most people. Stool passes through the anus and no permanent stoma is necessary; patient usually has temporary ileostomy while reservoir heals.

ILEOANAL RESERVOIR. With an ileoanal pull-through, the construction of an internal pouch, made of ileum, to provide some storage area for stool. Depending on how the ileum is looped before it is cut, folded and stitched to make the pouch, the reservoir is called a J-pouch (intestine with one loop, like the letter "J", the most common), An S-pouch, or a W-pouch.

ILEORECTAL ANASTAMOSIS. A surgical procedure in which the colon is removed, and the ileum is attached directly to the rectum.

ILEOSTOMY. Surgical opening into the ileum.

Conventional ileostomy (Brooke ileostomy). Intestine is severed and the end of the ileum is brought through the abdominal wall to form stoma, usually on the lower right side of abdomen. Entire colon and rectum is removed or bypassed. Pouch is worn over stoma at all times.

Continent ileostomy. See CONTINENT ILEOSTOMY.

Loop ileostomy. See LOOP OSTOMY.

INCONTINENCE. The inability to control passage of urine or stool.

INDIANA POUCH. See CONTINENT UROSTOMY.

INFLAMMATORY BOWEL DISEASE (IBD). Term for Crohn's disease and ulcerative colitis.

INTERMITTENT CATHETERIZATION. A technique used by people with urinary incontinence to empty the bladder at regular intervals by inserting a catheter through the urethra into the bladder.

INTRAVENOUS PYELOGRAM (IVP, excretory urography). Special x-rays of urinary tract. Medicine is injected into the vein so the urinary tract will show up clearly in the x-rays. (Not done if patient is allergic to iodine.)

IRRIGATION. For colostomates, an enema through the stoma of sigmoid or descending colostomy, done at regular intervals (usually every one-two days) to regulate the passage of stool. Water stretches the bowel, stimulates bowel to constrict and pass stool. One way of managing sigmoid or descending colostomy so person needs only gauze pad or security pouch over stoma between irrigations.

J-POUCH. See ILEOANAL RESERVOIR.

KARAYA. Water-soluble, gummy substance from the bark of a tree, used for healing or preventing damage to skin. Comes in gelatinous sheets, powder, paste; used as skin barrier around stoma.

LACTOSE INTOLERANCE. A deficiency of the enzyme lactase, needed for digestion of the sugar lactose found in dairy products. Frequently experienced by adults, leading to bloating, cramping and diarrhea when dairy products are consumed.

LOOP OSTOMY. One kind of stoma, usually for a temporary ostomy. Loop of intestine is brought through abdominal wall to form stoma; for several days, a plastic rod or "bridge" of tissue from the body under the loop keeps it from falling back into the abdomen. Loop is opened to create a single stoma with two openings. One opening, still connected to the food-digesting intestinal tract, continues to discharge stool; the other opening may discharge a small amount of mucus. Similar urinary tract ostomy can be made with ureter(s).

MAGNETIC RESONANCE IMAGING (MRI). An imaging technique which uses radiowaves to give cross-sectional pictures of internal body structures. Can be used to picture the urinary tract and the non-moving structures in the abdomen. For the patient, it involves lying still inside a large tube.

MONOCLONAL ANTIBODIES (MAbs). Laboratory-grown copies of the proteins produced by some of the body's defender cells. Research continues on using MAbs both for diagnosis and treatment of cancer.

MUCOUS FISTULA. With a temporary ostomy, the opening on the abdomen of the bypassed, non-functional segment of intestine. Since it is no longer connected to the food-digesting part of the intestinal tract, the mucous fistula does not excrete any stool but may still discharge some mucus. The mucous fistula can be the second of two stomas in a double-barrel ostomy, or the second opening in a single loop ostomy stoma. (Note: *mucous* is the adjective; *mucus* the noun.)

MUCUS. Fluid produced by the body to lubricate the digestive tract. Urinary tract ostomies which use a segment of the intestine continue to produce mucus, which appears in the urine.

NEPHROSTOMY. A temporary urinary diversion in which a plastic catheter (nephrostomy tube) is inserted through the skin into the kidney, stitched in place, and left to drain urine. The rest of the urinary tract is bypassed.

NIGHT DRAINAGE SYSTEM. Large container with tubing which can be connected to valve bottom of urostomy pouch at night or while the person is on bedrest.

Commercially-available or homemade systems provide additional storage capacity for urine; they keep pouches from becoming too full and pulling loose from the skin, and they keep urine draining away from the stoma.

NITRAZINE PAPER. Strips of paper which change color to show how acidic or alkaline urine is.

OBSTRUCTION (blockage). Any blockage in the digestive or urinary tract. Ileostomy obstruction often comes from insufficiently-chewed, high-cellulose foods (food blockage). Symptoms include no ostomy output over several hours, or spurts of watery stool, combined with abdominal cramping and nausea.

ONCOLOGIST. A doctor who specializes in the treatment of cancer (usually either medical or radiation oncologist).

OSTOMATE (Ostomist, in some countries). One name for the person who has a colostomy, ileostomy, or urinary ostomy.

OSTOMY. Surgical opening. Shortened name for colostomy, ileostomy, or urostomy.

OSTOMY VISITOR. Person with an ostomy, member of United Ostomy Association, who has completed a training program and visits people before or shortly after ostomy surgery. The visitor gives support and practical advice rather than medical information.

PATCH TESTING. Way of discovering whether a part of the ostomy pouching system causes allergic reaction. Small bit of product is taped on skin away from stoma area. Site is checked in 48 hours for redness, itching, swelling, and again 48 hours later for any delayed reaction. If symptoms occur earlier, product should be removed then.

PENILE IMPLANT. Semi-rigid rods or inflatable cylinders which can be surgically implanted in penis of a male who is unable to achieve or maintain erection.

PERINEAL WOUND (Posterior wound). Large gap where anus used to be. Occurs when rectum and anus are removed in colostomy or ileostomy surgery. Heals slowly as new tissue fills area. Can be closed, loosely stitched, or left open by surgeon.

PERISTALSIS. Normal progressive movement of intestine by which food, digestive enzymes and waste are pushed toward outlet (anus or stoma).

PERISTOMAL SKIN. Skin around the stoma.

PERMANENT OSTOMY. Ostomy meant to last through rest of person's lifetime. Additionally, a digestive tract ostomy in which the rectum and anus are removed, or a urinary tract ostomy in which the bladder is removed.

pH. How acid or alkaline substance is, compared to water.

POUCH (appliance, bag). Device worn over stoma to collect feces or urine. Pouches may be disposable or reusable, one- or two-piece, precut or cut-to-fit. They may have an attached skin barrier. They have different bottoms (valve, drainable, or closed-end), and are made of various materials in several shapes and sizes.

POUCHITIS. Inflammation of internal reservoir (either continent ileostomy or ileoanal anastomosis reservoir) causing pain, bloating and watery diarrhea. Treated with antibiotics.

PROCTOCOLECTOMY. See COLOPROCTECTOMY.

PROGNOSIS. Expected outcome of disease or other event.

PROLAPSE OF STOMA. Extreme protrusion ("falling out") of stoma end of intestine, an uncommon complication after ostomy surgery. The prolapsed stoma may protrude several inches from the body. This can be surgically corrected, if necessary.

REGIONAL ENTERITIS. See CROHN'S DISEASE.

REMISSION. The disappearance of all or most of the signs and symptoms of a cancer or other chronic disease. This can be for a period of time or permanent.

RESECTION. Cutting out section of intestine or other internal organ.

RETRACTED STOMA. Stoma below skin level.

REVISION. Construction of a new stoma/ostomy when the original one does not function well.

SIGMOID COLOSTOMY. See COLOSTOMY.

SIGMOIDOSCOPY. Visual examination of the anus, rectum, sigmoid colon and part of descending colon with 10-inch (25 cm) or longer lighted tube, either rigid or flexible. Biopsy specimens can be removed through the sigmoidoscope.

SKIN BARRIER. Any one of several substances (pliable

sheets, powders, pastes) used to cover skin around stoma to protect it from feces or urine.

SKIN SEALANT (Skin protectant). Liquids wiped, painted, or sprayed on the peristomal skin to protect the surface layer of skin cells. (Not a substitute for skin barrier.)

SMALL BOWEL SYNDROME. Condition in which not enough of small intestine remains to absorb nutrients necessary to sustain life. Can occur with Crohn's disease after surgical removal of large segment(s) of small intestine.

SPHINCTER. Ring-like muscle which opens and closes a body passageway. Two sphincters in anus provide bowel control; bladder sphincter controls urine.

STENOSIS (Stricture). Narrowing, often at opening of a stoma, so passage of stool or urine is partially or completely blocked. May need surgical correction.

STENT. A thin plastic tube used to keep narrow body passageways open while they heal after surgery (e.g., the connection between ureters and the segment of ileum in an ileal conduit). They are removed after healing is established.

STOMA. Visible portion of ostomy located on abdomen. A piece of ileum, colon, or ureter protruding above the skin.

TEMPORARY OSTOMY. A digestive tract ostomy in which the rectum and anus have not been removed or a urinary tract ostomy in which the bladder has not been removed.

TOTAL PARENTERAL NUTRITION (TPN, hyperalimentation). Administration of a nutritionally-adequate solution into a large vein, usually in the chest (central
intravenous line). Solution contains high-concentration
carbohydrate, protein, vitamins and minerals; fats can
also be given. A less concentrated solution can be given
through a smaller vein, usually in the arm (peripheral
parenteral nutrition, PPN).

TRANSVERSE COLOSTOMY. See COLOSTOMY.

ULCERATIVE COLITIS. One of the inflammatory bowel
diseases, in which ulcers form in the surface lining of
the colon and rectum. Severe, often bloody, diarrhea
is the primary symptom of this chronic disease, which
comes and goes unpredictably, and is experienced most
often by children, young adults and people over 60.
Removal of the colon and at least the surface layer of
the rectum is curative in severe cases. The cause of the
disease is unknown.

UNDIVERSION. Reconnection of the urinary tract after a
urinary diversion in which the bladder remains, to
eliminate the stoma and permit passage of urine
through the normal opening.

URETEROSTOMY. Ostomy procedure in which one or
both ureters are brought through the abdominal wall
to form stoma(s), often a loop ostomy. A temporary
procedure (unless the bladder is removed), frequently
performed on children. A pouch must be worn at all
times.

URINARY DIVERSION. Any one of several surgical procedures to reroute urine flow away from diseased or
defective ureters, bladder or urethra, either temporarily

or permanently. Some diversions result in a stoma. See COLONIC CONDUIT, CONTINENT UROSTOMY, ILEAL CONDUIT, NEPHROSTOMY, URETEROSTOMY, VESICOSTOMY.

URINARY KOCK POUCH. See CONTINENT UROSTOMY.

URINARY TRACT. Body organs which make, transport, store and eliminate urine. Urine is made in the two *kidneys*, passes from each kidney down a narrow tube (*ureter*) to a single expandable storage chamber (*bladder*), and from there is passed outside the body through a single tube (*urethra*).

URINE CRYSTALS. Sharp, gritty crystals which can encrust on a urostomy stoma or unprotected peristomal skin. See ENCRUSTATION.

UROSTOMY. Any kind of urinary diversion which results in a stoma. New passageway for urine is formed through abdominal wall to outside the body. See URINARY DIVERSION.

VESICOSTOMY. A temporary urinary diversion (rarely done now) in which the bladder opens directly to a stoma, located low on the abdomen. Some are drained with a catheter.

INDEX

Abdominoperineal (A-P)
   resection, 74, 76, 93, 291.
   See also Colostomy,
      Ileostomy
Absenteeism, 233.
   See also Disability, Work
Acceptance
   and employment, 234
   of ostomy experience, 63-66
   of temporary ostomy, 158
   See also Attitude, Emotions
Activity. See Employment,
   Exercise, Ostomy, Sports
Adhesive remover, 137
Adhesives, 52, 125-26, 137, 141
Adrenal glands, and stress,
   173, 174, 176
Airplane travel, 258-60
Alcohol
   and diet, 166
   and sex, 187
Alimentary canal. See
   Digestive tract
Allergies
   to ostomy products, 119, 121
   patch testing for, 121, 143,
      304-5
   See also Skin
Alterescu, Victor, RN, ET, 63,
   65-66, 119
Alvers, Jean, ET, 53, 208, 262
American Cancer Society
   (ACS), 253, 268, 280, 289
American Hospital
   Association, 28
American Journal of Nursing, 266
Americans with Disabilities
   Act of 1990, 234, 238

Anastomosis, 74, 96, 291.
   See also Ileoanal
      anastomosis, Ileorectal
      anastomosis
Anatomy of an Illness
   (Cousins), 176
Anesthesia
   general, 44
   aftereffects of, 48-49
Anger
   of family, 210, 287
   after surgery, 8, 158.
   See also Acceptance,
      Attitude, Emotions
Anti-reflux valve, 106, 107,
   109, 291, 295.
   See also Urine, Urostomy
Antibiotics
   and bowel prep, 292
   for inflammatory bowel
      disease, 89
   pre-surgery, 40.
   See also Medicine
Anus
   abscesses around, 88
   and digestion, 18
   maintenance of, 97
   removal of, 5, 7, 73, 74-75,
      76, 93
   for urinary diversion, 107
   See also Colostomy,
      Digestive tract, Ileoanal
      anastomosis, Ileorectal
      anastomosis, Ileostomy,
      Perineal wound, Rectum
Anxiety
   about sex, 187, 194.
   See also. Sex

A-P resection. See
   Abdominoperineal
   resection
Appliances for stoma
   See Pads, Pouches
Artificial anus surgery, 73.
   See also Colostomy
Artificial urinary sphincter, 108
Ascending colostomy.
   See Colostomy
Attitude
   and healing from grief, 60,
   63-66
   effect of on healing
   process, 27-28, 71-72
   about temporary ostomies,
   146-47, 157-59, 160-62.
   See also Acceptance,
   Emotions, Body Image,
   Self Image
Auto-immune disease
   and inflammatory bowel
   disease, 89
Automobile travel, 258
Autonomy
   of children, 209
   in managing stoma, 53-54
   patient, 26-41
   after surgery, 9

Bag bulge, 129, 169.
   See also Gas, Pouches
Baking soda
   for cleaning peristomal skin,
   138
   for electrolyte replacement,
   165
Barium enema/x-ray, 36, 88,
   291
   small bowel, 222-24, 291
   See also Bowel prep, Tests,
   X-ray
Basketball, 249

Bathing, 25
   after irrigation, 85
   and sex appeal, 192-93
Bathroom needs
   and employment, 234
   and travel, 253, 256-57, 258
   See also Privacy
BCG vaccine, 228
Belts, for pouches, 142
Berenstein, Natalie, 205
Berry, Don, 230
Bile, in stool, 76
Bills, medical: right to explanation of, 32
Binder, Don, 122, 275, 276-77
Biofeedback, 178
Biological therapy, 225-26,
   227-28
   side effects of, 228
Biopsy, 2, 36, 88, 224, 292, 293
Birth control pills, 197
Birth defects, ostomies for,
   205-6, 214. See also Familial
   polyposis, Gardner's
   Syndrome
Bladder
   biopsy of, 36
   infection of, 58
   internal substitutes for, 106-7
   normal role of, 20, 102
   pacemaker for, 108
   removal/bypass of, 5-6, 14,
   103-4.
   See also Cancer, Cystectomy, Nephrostomy,
   Ureterostomy, Urinary
   diversion, Urinary tract,
   Urostomy, Vesicostomy
Bleeding. See Bowel, Skin,
   Stoma
Blockage, 19, 98, 168, 304
   from barium, 223-24
Blood tests, pre-surgery, 37

Body hair
    and pouches, 139, 299
    and pre-surgery shaving, 43
Body image
    and clothing, 181
    after surgery, 8, 61, 158.
        See also Body image,
        Clothing, Self image
Bolinger, Bonnie, RN, ET,
    267-68
Boston Ostomy Association,
    262-63
Bowel
    bleeding from, 3, 20
    changes in, 3, 20, 64.
        See also Anus, Colon, Diges-
        tive tract, Feces, Inflam-
        matory bowel disease,
        Peristalsis, Rectum, Stool
Bowel prep, 35-36, 39-40, 108,
    292
    with ostomy, 222-24
Breathing
    and stress management, 176
    after surgery, 44-45.
        See also Lung complications
Brewer, Bobbie, 265
Bricker, Dr., 104
Bricker loop. See Ileal conduit
Brooke, Bryan, M.D., 91
Brooke ileostomy procedure,
    91, 94, 301.
        See also Ileostomy
Brown, John Young, M.D., 91
Bullock, Wynn, 65

Calories, 166
Cameron, Gerry, RN, ET, 268
Camping, 256-57, 259
Canadian Association for Enteros-
    tomal Therapy, 270, 289
Canadian Cancer Society
    (CCS), 289

Cancer
    and attitude, 229
    of bladder, 20, 57, 101, 107,
        226, 228
    of colon, 5, 19, 30, 33, 35,
        57, 74-75, 97, 146, 226-
        27, 228, 292
    and diet, 167, 170
    and discrimination in
        employment, 238
    and eating, 163
    feelings about, 64-65
    and fertility, 197
    and pregnancy, 200
    preventing recurrence of,
        57, 221-24
    of rectum, 2, 4, 14, 64, 74
    resources on, 229
    and sex, 195
    and stress, 174
    and support, 229
    tests for, 221-24
    treatment for, 225-29.
        See also Barium enema/
        x-ray, Biological therapy,
        Chemotherapy, Familial
        polyposis, Gardner's
        Syndrome, Radiation
        therapy
Carbohydrates, 163
Carbonated drinks, 169
Carcinogenic-embryonic
    Antigen (CEA), 221, 292
Care, right to continuity of, 32
Carroll, Lewis, 162
Catheter
    for continent ileostomy, 98
    post-surgery, 47, 58
    for urinary incontinence, 108
        See also Intermittent
        catheterization
Cecostomy, 151-52, 155,
    292

Cecum, 292
  in urostomy, 106
  See also Cecostomy
Cellulose, 168. *See also* Fiber
Chaplains, hospital, 29
Check-ups, 220-20
  anxiety about, 221
  frequency of, 229-30
  and stoma, 222-24
  for urostomy, 111
  See also Cancer, Hospitals
Cheerleading, 245
Chemotherapy, for cancer, 57,
    107, 225, 226-27
  ambulatory pumps for, 227
  side effects of, 227
  See also Cancer
Chewing, of food, 168-69
Children, of parents with
    ostomies, 72
Children, with ostomy, 205-12
  acceptance of, 210-11
  autonomy of, 209
  care of, 208-9
  and clothing, 184
  examples of, 205-7
  and friends, 211
  parents of, 210
  preschoolers, 205, 208-9
  reasons for, 205-6
  and school, 211
  stomas of, 109
  and support, 211-12, 280
  with temporary ostomy,
    206, 209
  with urostomy, 14, 103, 152
  See also Teenager
Cholesterol, 166-67
Chris has an Ostomy (United
    Ostomy Association), 208
Claitman, Ed, 235-36
Clinical trials, for cancer
    treatments, 229.

See also Experimentation
Clothing, 180-85
  after convalescence, 182-85
  during convalescence, 180,
    181-82
  low budget, 183
  for travel, 254
Colectomy, 93, 292.
  See also Colon, Colostomy,
  Ileostomy
Colitis. See Ulcerative colitis
Colon
  ascending, 107
  descending, 206
  and digestion, 18-19, 75-76
  removal/rerouting of, 5, 13,
    93 *See also* Bowels, Can-
    cer, Colostomy, Digestive
    tract, Ileostomy, Inflam-
    matory bowel disease
Colonic conduit, 21, 104, 106,
  292-93. *See also* Ileal
  conduit, Urostomy
Colonoscopy, 35, 88, 293
  through stoma, 224
Coloproctectomy, 93, 293
Colorectal cancer. See Cancer
Colostomies—A Guide
  (United Ostomy
  Association), 53-54
Colostomy, 2, 5, 13, 19, 73-85,
  291, 293-94
  ascending, 293
  and cancer treatments, 226
  and check-ups for cancer,
    222-24
  descending, 54, 294
  determining type of, 74-77
  examples of persons with,
    14, 15
  history of techniques for, 73-74
  longevity with, 74
  lumbar, 73

Colostomies (cont.)
  need for, 19-20, 74-75
  and perineal wound, 54-56
  post-surgery, 47
  prevalence of, 14, 19
  sigmoid, 54, 76, 77, 78, 118,
    193, 243, 294
  stoma of, 23
  surgical procedures for, 20,
    74-76
  temporary, 15, 19, 33, 75,
    145
  transverse, 293, 308
  and travel, 253, 256-57
  See also Irrigation, Ostomy,
    Pouches, Stoma, Surgery,
    Temporary
    ostomy
Colostomy plug, 118, 125
  and irrigation, 78
  for short periods, 80, 193,
    243
Computed tomography
  (CT scan), 294
  and cancer testing, 222
  and pre-surgery testing, 37
Confidentiality, right to, 31
Connors, Melba, 266-67, 272
Consent, informed, 30-31
Constipation
  causes of, 81
  remedies for, 80-81
Consumer Information Center,
  289
Continent intestinal reservoir
  (CIR). See Ileostomy
  (continent)
Continent ostomy. See Ostomy
Continent urostomy.
  See Urostomy
Conventional ileostomy. See
  Brooke ileostomy
  procedure, Ileostomy

Convexity
  in pouch system, 126-27,
    295
Coughing
  after surgery, 44-45
  See also Breathing, Lung
    complications
Counseling, professional, 66,
  175, 189, 192, 194.
  See also Enterostomal-
    therapy nurses
Cousins, Norma, 175-76
Cramping, abdominal
  from inflammatory bowel
    disease, 87, 89
  from intestinal blockage, 168
  during irrigation, 84
  from pouchitis, 96
Cranberry juice, for urine
  encrustation, 111-12
Crohn's and Colitis Founda-
  tion of America, Inc.
  (CCFA), 89, 239, 289
Crohn's disease, 5, 87-88, 90,
  295
  surgery for, 96-97
  teenagers with, 213
  See also Fistulas, Inflam-
    matory bowel disease
Crying, 62, 63. *See also*
  Emotions, Grieving
CT scan. See Computed
  tomography
Cystectomy, 103-4, 295. *See
  also* Bladder, Urostomy
Cystoscopy, 36, 108, 296
Cystostomy, 103.
  See also Urostomy

Dairy products
  allergy to, 90, 169, 302
  milk, 163, 164
  See also Lactose intolerance

Dancing, 246
Davis, Lawrence P., M.D., 197
Defecate, urge to, 56
Dehydration
    and activity, 233, 248
    and inflammatory bowel
        disease, 90
    during travel, 255, 256,
        258-59
    See also Fluids, Water
Deodorants, 129
Depression
    after surgery, 8
    and sex, 187
Descending colostomy. See
    Colostomy
Diabetes, 170
Diarrhea
    and diet, 79
    and inflammatory bowel
        disease, 20, 87, 89
    and travel, 255
    See also Stool, loose
Diet, 162-71
    and bowel control, 79-80
    and gas, 79, 169-70
    for ileostomy, 167-78
    for inflammatory bowel
        disease, 89-90
    liquid, 39, 90
    and odor, 129
    special needs and, 164-65
    after surgery, 49, 51, 162-63,
        168
    before surgery, 34, 35, 39, 40
    starvation, 35
    and travel, 255.
    See also Fiber, Nutrients
Digestive Diseases National
    Coalition (DDNC), 280
Digestive tract, 296
    adjustment of after surgery,
        47, 71, 99, 158

breakdown in, 19
    with colostomy, 76
    normal process of, 15-19, 75-76
    and stress, 173, 175
Disability insurance, 58-59
Discharge planner. See Social
    worker/discharge planner
Discrimination, in
    employment, 238
Dreams, stoma in, 25
Driving, 233
Dubin, Sam, 275
    Achievement Award, 276

ECG. See Electrocardiogram
Ejaculation, failure of, 187,
    194, 196-97. *See also* Sex
EKG. See Electrocardiogram
Electrocardiogram, 37
Electrodes, in recovery room, 45
Electrolytes, 164-65, 256, 297.
    See also Minerals, Potas-
    sium, Sodium
Emergency alert emblem,
    254-55
Emerson, Ralph Waldo, 132
Emotions, 8, 60-66
    in adjusting to life, 67-68
    over body image, 61
    about children, 210, 216
    and excretory function, 61
    and feeling different, 62
    of partner, 191-92
    and temporary ostomies,
        157-59.
    See also Acceptance, Anger,
    Attitude, Body image,
    Children, Depression,
    Family, Grieving, Self
    image, Teenagers
Employers, dealing with,
    233-34

Employment, 231-240
and ability, 231-33
application for, 236-38
and changing careers, 235
and discrimination, 236-38
and employees, 234
and employers, 233-34
and openness, 234, 235-36
and special needs, 234
See also Disability, Sick leave
Encrustation, urine 111-12, 119, 297
Endoscopy, 88, 297. *See also* Colonoscopy, Cystoscopy, Sigmoidoscopy
Enemas, for bowel prep, 36, 39. *See also* Bowel prep, Irrigation
Enterostomal therapists, 8. *See also* Enterostomal therapy nurses
Enterostomal therapy, 8, 261-72
origins of, 261-63
See also Enterostomal therapy nurses
Enterostomal therapy nurses (ET nurses), 8-9, 14, 262, 297-98
certified (CETNs), 264, 298
for emotional support, 265
in foreign countries, 270-71
and job satisfaction, 272
for locating stoma site, 24, 40, 265
prevalence of, 265
qualifications for, 263-264, 265-66
responsibilities of, 264-65
scholarships for, 270
for sex information, 194
for teaching stoma care, 53, 264

training for, 269-70
See also Enterostomal therapy
Enterostomy, 14, 298. *See also* Ostomy
Enzymes, and skin care, 99, 117, 119, 154. *See also* Skin
Erection, failure of, 187, 194-96. *See also* Sex
Esophagus, 15
ET nurses. See Enterostomal therapy nurses
Excoriation, 298. *See also* Skin
Excretory urography. See Intravenous pyelogram
Exercise, 241-49
and stress management, 176, 244
and taking it easy, 243-44, 248
See also Activity, Jogging, Perspiration, Sports, Swimming, Walking
Expense, of ostomy equipment, 130
Experimentation, and treatment, 32. *See also* Clinical trials

Faceplates, of pouches, 125-26, 141. *See also* Pouches
Facing Forward: A Guide for Cancer Survivors (HHS), 238
Familial polyposis, 97, 295, 298
and pregnancy, 200
Family, 283-88
grieving of, 62, 286-87
as part of treatment team, 29
support of, 58, 175
See also Children, Parents
Fast-dividing cells, 227
Fatigue
from cancer treatment, 226, 227

Fatigue (cont.)
  after surgery, 10, 70-71
Fats, 163
  reduction of, 164, 166
Feces, 18, 299
  formation of, 75-76
  See also Stool
Feelings. See Anger, Attitude,
  Body image, Depression,
  Emotions, Grieving
Fencing, 246
Fiber, dietary, 166-69
  and bowel regulation, 79, 167
  for colostomy, 167
  for ileostomy, 167-68
  and inflammatory bowel
    disease, 89-90
Fields, W. C., 186
Fistulas, caused by Crohn's
  disease, 88, 199. *See also*
  Mucous fistula
Fletcherism, 168-69
Fluids, need for:
  with ileostomy, 99, 165
  during pregnancy, 202
  during travel, 255
  with urostomy, 110, 165.
  See also Diet, Water
Flush stoma. See Stoma
Folliculitis, 299. *See also* Body
  hair
Food. See Chewing, Diet,
  Fiber, Nutrients
Friends
  grief of, 62
  as part of treatment team, 29
  reactions of, 10
  support of, 58, 175
  and temporary ostomy, 161.
  See also Family, Sex

Gall bladder, 15
Gallstones, 99, 170

Gambrell, Ed, 78-79, 234
Gardner's Syndrome, 97, 299.
  See also Cancer (colon)
Gas
  causes of, 169
  and diet, 79, 169-70
  and ileostomy, 98
  and pouches, 125, 128-30, 170
  remedies for, 169-70
  as warning sign of cancer, 20
Gaskell, Eunice, RN, ET, 268-69
Gastrostomy tube, 47
Gay and Lesbian Concerns
  Committee of UOA, 197, 280
Geddes, Barbara Bel, 58
Geiger, Virginia Pearce, 277
Gelernt, Irwin, M.D., 203
General Assistance, 59
Gill, Norma, 261-62, 276
Ginger, to relieve post-surgery
  nausea 51
Golfing, 244
Granulomatous disease of the
  bowel. See Crohn's disease
Greaves, Judy, 38
Grieving
  and family, 62, 287
  and letting go, 63-64, 65-66
  sharing of, 62-63
  for organs of elimination, 61
  with temporary ostomy,
    158-59
  See also Acceptance,
    Attitude, Depression,
    Emotions
Gut. See Digestive tract
Gymnastics, 245-46

Hartmann's pouch, 150, 151,
  299. *See also* Temporary ostomy
Hastings, Robert J., 144

Health care professionals
patient's partnership with,
27-29, 228-29
on treatment team, 29-30
See also Hospitals, Pregnancy, Oncologists,
Urologists
Health insurance, 58, 59, 239-40
for international travel, 260
Heat. See Dehydration,
Perspiration
Heavy lifting, ability to do, 233
Hedgepeth, William, 172
Help for Incontinent People
(HIP), 108, 290
Hernia, 224, 300
Hertel, Norbert, 86
High blood pressure, 170
and stress, 173
Hobbies, and stress management, 176
Hockey, 244
Holistic health movement, 27
Homosexuals, in United Ostomy Association. See Gay
and Lesbian Concerns Committee
Honesty. See Openness
Horseback riding, 247
Hospitals
discharge from, 10, 58-59, 67
ostomy supplies to bring to,
225
and patient's rights, 31, 32
and preparation for surgery,
34
and staff ignorance, 222-23,
224-25
teaching, 32, 37
and visitors, 37-38, 58, 214
See also Health care professionals, Pregnancy, Social
worker/discharge

planner, Surgery
Humor, 62, 176. *See also*
Attitude
Huxley, Aldous, 177
Hyperalimentation, 90
Hyperplasia, 111, 300. *See also*
Stoma, Urostomy

Ileal conduit, 20-21, 104-5,
300. *See also* Urostomy
Ileal pouch-anal anastomosis.
See Ileoanal anastomosis
Ileal reservoir, 95-96. See
Ileoanal anastomosis,
Ileoanal reser voir,
Urostomy
Ileitis. See Crohn's disease
Ileoanal anastomosis, 96. *See
also* Ileoanal reservoir
Ileoanal pull-through procedure, 96, 300. *See also* Ileal
reser voir, Ileoanal reservoir
Ileoanal reservoir, 95, 300-301.
See also Ileal reservoir,
Ileoanal anastomosis
Ileorectal anastomosis, 96, 97,
298, 301
in teenagers, 217-18
Ileostomy, 5, 13-14, 86-100,
291, 301
and activity (physical), 233,
240-41, 244, 245-46
and blockage, 168
and clothing, 183, 184
continent, 93, 94, 203, 294-95
and dietary fiber, 167-68
and drinking fluids, 165
getting used to, 98-100
history of, 91, 93
and ileal anastamosis
surgery, 95-96
need for, 20, 86-91, 97

Ileostomy (cont.)
  and perineal wound, 54-56,
    98
  post-surgery, 47, 98-99
  prevalence of, 20
  and remission, 88
  special problems of, 99-100
  stoma of, 23, 91, 93, 99-100
  support for patients, 97-98
  surgical procedures for, 20,
    93-97
  temporary, 15, 19, 96, 145,
    217-18
  and travel, 251, 255, 256,
    259-60
  and weight gain, 166
  See also Ileal reservoir,
    Ileoanal reservoir, Os-
    tomy, Temporary ostomy
Ileostomy Association of New
  York, 246
The Ileostomy Quartery, 262-
  63, 275. See also Ostomy
  Quarterly
Ileum, 5, 13-14
  role of in digestion, 75-76
  use of in urostomy, 21,
    104, 106
  See also Digestive tract,
    Ileostomy
Immune system
  and biological therapy, 227-28
  and inflammatory bowel
    disease, 89
Incision, abdominal
  healing of, 51
  pain of, 48
  stitches of, 7
  in surgery, 74
  See also Perineal wound
Incontinence, 101, 107-8, 301
  in children, 206, 207

See also Urinary tract diversion, Urine, Urostomy
Indiana pouch, 106-7. See also
  Ileostomy (continent), Urostomy (continent)
Infection
  post-operative, 39
  signs of, 57, 58
  See also Bladder, Kidneys,
    Urinary tract
Inflammatory bowel disease
  (IBD), 14-15, 19, 20, 86-97,
    103
  and barium x-rays, 36, 88
  diagnosis of, 88
  nonsurgical treatment for,
    89-90
  nutrition for, 89-90
  occurence of, 88-89
  and pre-surgery building
    up, 34, 98
  and re-employment, 233,
    236-37
  and stress, 174
  teenagers with, 215
  types of, 89-90
  See also Crohn's disease,
    Ileostomy, Ulcerative
    colitis
Information, patient rights to,
  28, 30-31, 32. See also Rights
Inherited diseases, ileostomy
  for, 97. See also Birth
  defects, Familial polyposis,
  Gardner's Syndrome
Insurance. See Disability insurance, Health insurance
Intercourse, painful, 194. See
  also Erection, Sex
Interferons, 228
Interleukins, 228
Intermittent catheterization,
  108, 301

International Association for Enterostomal Therapy (IAET), 253, 263, 265, 269, 270, 290

International Association for Medical Assistance to Travelers (IAMAT), 260, 290

International Ostomy Association, 254, 271, 280, 290

Intestinal system. See Digestive tract

Intravenous (IV) line, 46
and inflammatory bowel disease, 90, 98

Intravenous pyelogram (IVP), 36, 108, 111, 222, 301-2

Irrigating clips, 82, 85

Irrigating cone, 82, 84, 85, 294

Irrigating dam, 84

Irrigating sleeve, 82, 84, 85

Irrigating tip, 84, 85

Irrigating tube, 82, 83

Irrigating water-flow clamp, 82, 83

Irrigation, 21, 302
alternatives to, 54, 79-80
for barium enema/x-ray, 223
description of, 78-79
and gas, 170
methods for, 78-79, 82-85
pros and cons of, 53-54, 76
in temporary colostomy, 154
and travel, 252, 258

Irrigation kit, 82
cleaning of, 85

IVP. See Intravenous pyelogram

J-pouch, 96, 301. *See also* Ileoanal reservoir

Jet lag, and regulation, 258-59

Jeter, Katherine F., ET, 101, 118

Jobs. See Employment

Jogging, 241-42

Journal of the American Medical Association, 274

Journal of ET Nursing, 63, 270

Julian, Margot, RN, ET, 271-71

Junk foods, 166. *See also* Diet

Karaya, 120, 243, 302

Karon, Ira, 274

Kidney stones, 99, 170

Kidneys
compensation of, 165
and ileostomy, 99
infection of, 102, 104, 109, 110-11, 206
role of, 20, 102
and urostomy, 102, 104, 109
See also Urinary tract

Klein, Elsie, 64-65

Kock, Nils, 94, 106

Kock pouch
for ileostomy, 94, 294
for urostomy, 106, 295
See also Ileostomy (continent), Urostomy (continent)

Lactose intolerance, 90, 169, 302

Laissez-faire approach, to bowel management, 80. *See also* Colostomy, Pouches

Large intestine, 296. *See also* Anus, Colon, Digestive tract, Rectum

Laxatives
for bowel prep, 36, 39
for constipation, 81
for travel, 253

Lenneberg, Edith, 262-64, 281

Letting go. See Acceptance, Grieving

Lingerie, 182, 193. *See also* Clothing
Litmus. See Nitrazine paper
Litwack, Larry, 282
Liver, 15
Loneliness, 68
Longevity, with ostomy surgery, 74
Loop ostomy. See Ostomy
Loss, sense of. See Grieving
Lung complications
 prevention of, 38, 44-45
 See also Breathing, Coughing
Lying
 about feeling bad, 62
 See also Emotions, Openness
Lyons, Albert S., M.D., 199, 274

Magnetic resonance imaging (MRI), 37, 303
Marathon running, 244-45
Mau, Marilyn, 279
McGuire, Dolores E., 198
Medicine
 and constipation, 81
 for inflammatory bowel disease, 89
 for erection problems, 196
 with ileostomy, 100
 for post-surgical pain, 46
 and sex, 187
 and travel, 253
 See also Anesthesia, Antibiotics
Meditation, 177
Memory loss, after anesthesia, 48-49
Men
 problems with sex of, 187, 194-97
 urinary diversion for, 107

Metro Maryland newsletter, 181
Metro Maryland Youth Ostomy Association, 213
Miles, William Ernest, M.D., 74
Minerals, 163, 164. *See also* Electrolytes, Potassium, Sodium
Modeling, with ostomy pouch, 183-84
Monoclonal antibodies (MAbs), 221-22, 228, 303
Morley, Christopher, 1
Mouth, and digestion, 15
MRI tests. See Magnetic resonance imaging
Mucous fistula, 148, 150, 303
 care of, 154
 See also Ostomy (double-barrel, loop)
Mucus, 25, 111, 303
Muscles, abdominal,
 after surgery, 243
 in digestive tract, 18-19
 See also Peristalsis, Sphincter
Mutual aid groups. See Support groups

Nasogastric (NG) tube, 46-47
National Cancer Institute (NCI), 238
National Cancer Institute, Cancer Information Service, 170, 229
National Coalition for Cancer Survivorship (NCCS), 238, 290
Nausea
 during irrigation, 84
 post-surgery, 51
Neary, Lucy, 274
Nephrostomy, 103, 152, 155, 303. *See also* Urinary diversion, Urostomy

Night drainage system, 109-10, 303-4. *See also* Pouches, Sleep, Urostomy

Nightclothes, 182. *See also* Clothing

Nitrazine paper, 112, 304

Noise, from pouches, 129-30

Norris, Carol, 241-42, 259

Nudism, with ostomy pouch, 4-5

Nurses, 29
  recovery room, 43
  See also Enterostomal therapy nurses, Health care professionals

Nutrients, in food, 163-68
  absorption of, 19
  See also Diet, Digestive tract, Fiber, Minerals

Nutrition for the Chemotherapy Patient (Ramstack and Rosenbaum), 170

Obstruction. See Blockage

Odor
  and cleanliness, 119, 128
  with ileostomy, 98
  and pouches, 128-29, 170
  See also Gas, Pouches

Oncologist, 57, 228-29, 304

Openness
  and employment, 234, 235-38
  about feelings, 62-64
  about ostomy, 11-12, 69-70, 189-91
  See also Acceptance, Attitude, Emotions

Orgasm, problems of, 194. *See also* Sex

Ostomate Bill of Rights, 40, 42

Ostomate, definition of, 13, 304. *See also* Ostomy

Ostomy, 1, 13, 304
  and activity (physical), 4-5, 231-33, 241-49
  continent, 21-22, 94
  double-barrel, 150, 296-97
  and employment, 231-40
  end, 154, 297
  examples of persons with, 14-15, 27
  getting used to, 50-59, 60-66
  history of, 25
  loop, 148-50, 155, 302
  and patients' rights, 27-32
  permanent, 305
  prevalence of, 6
  reasons for, 19-20
  refusal of, 12
  temporary, 145
  and travel, 250-60
  types of, 5-6, 13-14
  See also Colostomy, Enterostomal therapy nurses, Ileostomy, Pouches, Stoma, Supplies, Surgery, Temporary ostomy, Urostomy

Ostomy Quarterly (United Ostomy Association), 69, 74, 122, 193, 253, 275, 277

Ostomy visitor, 304. *See also* United Ostomy Association

Oxygen, in recovery room, 45

Pads
  for stoma, 21, 24, 118
  with irrigation, 78
  with urostomy, 106

Pancreas, 15

Parents
  of children with ostomy, 210
  with ostomies, 72
  of teenagers with ostomies, 215-16

Parents (cont.)
 See also Children, Family,
  Teenagers
Patch test, for skin allergies,
 121, 143, 304-5. *See also* Al-
 lergies, Skin
Patient's Bill of Rights, 28, 30-32
Patient-Controlled Analgesia
 (PCA), 46
Pelvic pouch procedure. See
 Ileoanal anastomosis
Penile implants, 195, 305. *See
 also* Erection
Perineal wound, 48, 51, 305
 and clothing, 182
 healing of, 54-56, 98
 incision of, 74
 inspection of, 222
 and pregnancy, 202, 203
 sensations in, 56-57
 and sex, 194
 See also Incision
Perineum, 55. *See also*
 Perineal wound
Peripheral parenteral nutrition
 (PPN), 90
Peristalsis, 18-19, 305
 with urostomy, 104
Peristomal skin. See Skin
Perspiration
 and skin care, 119-20
 and sodium intake, 165
pH, 305. *See also* Urine
Pharmacological Erection
 Program (PEP), 196
Physical examinations. See
 Check-ups
Physicians. See Health care
 professionals, Oncologists,
 Pregnancy, Urologists
Planning, for future, 58-59
Plastic surgery, 194
Play therapy, for children, 208

Plug, colostomy. See Colostomy plug
Polyps. See Familial Polyposis,
 Gardner's Syndrome
Posterior wound. See Perineal
 wound
Potassium, 99, 165, 259-60
Pouches, 21, 109, 114-31, 132-
 43, 171, 305
 using adhesives for, 52, 125-
  26, 137, 141
 ad hoc, 114-15
 application of, 140-41
 changing of, 52-53, 135-43
 for children, 208-9
 choosing of, 122-28
 closing of, 132-33
 cleaning of, 123, 134, 142-43
 closed-end colostomy, 52
 under clothing, 182
 for colostomy, 118
 covers for, 123, 193, 258
 disposable, 123, 125, 139,
  203-4
 drainable, 52, 80, 116-8,
  132-34
 emptying of, 133-34
 and gas dispersal, 128-30
 history of, 115-16
 for ileostomy, 98, 100, 117
 for irregularly shaped
  stomas, 126
 with irrigation, 78
 and "laissez-faire" bowel
  management, 80
 leaks in, 135
 management of, 132-43
 non-adhesive, 126
 one-piece, 123
 during pregnancy, 202, 203-4
 as protection for stoma, 24
 removal of, 137-38
 reusable, 123, 125-26

Pouches (cont.)
  and sports, 248-49
  and swimming, 243
  using tape for, 141, 142, 143
  two-piece, 125
  types of, 116-18
  for urostomy, 6, 104, 108-9,
    113, 116
  See also Bag bulge, Exercise,
    Gas, Skin, Supplies, Travel
Pouchitis, 96, 305-6
Prayer, 177. *See also* Serenity
  Prayer
Pre-surgery, 33-42
  and bowel prep, 35-36
  tests of, 33-34, 35-37
  waiting period of, 33-34
  See also Bowel prep,
    Surgery
Pregnancy, 197, 198-204
  and Caesarian section, 203
  and delivery, 203-4
  and doctors, 200-201
  and hospital staff, 203
  prohibitions to, 200
  special needs for, 202-4
  timing of, 199-200
Preternatural anus surgery, 73.
  See also Colostomy
Privacy
  and irrigation, 79
  right to, 31
Proctocolectomy, 93. *See also*
  Coloproctectomy
Prognosis, 306
Project SHARE, 281
Prolapse of stoma. See Stoma
Proteins, 163, 164

QT New York, 274

Radiation therapy, for cancer,
  57, 75, 107, 225

side effects of, 226
stoma care during, 226. *See
  also* Cancer
Recovery room, 45. *See also*
  Hospitals, Surgery
Rectal cancer. See Cancer
Rectum
  and digestion, 18, 19
  removal of, 5, 74-75, 76, 93
  See also Cancer, Colostomy,
    Ileostomy, Perineal
    wound
Regional enteritis. See Crohn's
  disease
Relaxation
  and irrigation, 79
  and stress management,
    176-77
  techniques for, 177-78
  See also Stress
Remen, Naomi, M.D., 210, 214-15
Remission, 306. *See also* Cancer
Resection, 306
  of tumor, 74
  See also Abdominoperineal
    resection
Reservoir (internal pouch), 21-
  22. *See also* Ileal reservoir,
    Ileoanal reservoir
Respiratory therapists, 38
Responsibilities
  of patient, 27-28
  of physician, 26-27
  See also Autonomy, Rights
Retracted stoma. See Stoma
Revascularization surgery, 196.
  See also Erection
Revision. See Stoma
Rightman, David, 235
Rights, of patient, 28-32
Rosebud (nickname for
  stoma), 52
Ryan, Mary, 190-91

St. Paul's Colostomy and Ileos-
tomy Rehabilitation Guild,
Inc., 275-76
Salt. See Sodium
Santa Rosa News Herald, 69-70
School of Enterostomal
Therapy, 262
Schreiber, George, M.D., 274
Schreiber, Mike, 264
Secrecy, about ostomies, 11-
12. *See also* Openness
Self image, 175, 237, 245. *See
also* Acceptance, Attitude,
Body image, Clothing
Selye, Hans, 173
Serenity Prayer, 50, 175
Sex, with ostomy, 186-97
and communication, 188,
189-91, 193
emotions about, 186- 87
and fatigue, 187
and partner's reaction, 189,
191-92
and pouches, 193
problems of, 187, 194-97
and self-acceptance, 188-89
without intercourse, 196
Sexually-transmitted disease, 197
Shakespeare, William, 273
Sick leave, 58
Sigmoid colostomy. See
Colostomy
Sigmoidoscope, 2, 35
Sitz baths, 56
Skiing, 247
Skin barriers, 120-21, 125, 128,
306-7
application of, 139-40, 141
"extended wear", 135
fitting of, 136-37
paste for, 139, 140
and temperature extremes, 257
and temporary ostomy, 154-55

Skin, peristomal
care and cleaning of, 118-
21, 138, 154, 157
in children, 208
infection of, 120
irritation of, 99-100, 119-20,
111-12, 117, 135
protection of, 136-37.
See also Allergies, Pouches,
Skin barriers, Stoma
Skin sealants, 121, 307
Sleep, and stress management,
177
during travel, 254
with urostomy, 109-10, 303-4
See also Night drainage
system
Sleeping pills, 177
Slutzky, Dave, 277
Small bowel syndrome, 96,
307. *See also* Crohn's disease
Small intestine, 5, 18, 296. *See
also* Digestive tract, Ileum
Smoking, effects of on
surgery, 38
Social contact, and stress
management, 176-77. *See
also* Friends, Sex, Support,
Support groups
Social Security Administration,
59
Social worker/discharge plan-
ner, 58, 59
Sodium, 99, 165. *See also*
Electrolytes, Minerals
Sorrow. See Emotions
Sphincter muscles, 307
and colostomy, 74, 76
and digestion, 18
and ileorectal anastomosis,
97
See also Anus, Artificial
urinary sphincter, Bladder

Spina bifida, 247
Sports, 242-47
  getting started in, 247-49
  See also Basketball,
    Dancing, Exercise, Golf,
    Hockey, Horseback
    riding, Jogging, Swim-
    ming, Walking
Stair, Nadine, 178-79
Stenosis, 307. *See also* Blockage
Stents, 108, 307
Steroids, and surgery, 98
Stiches. See Incision, Peristomal wound
Stoma, 5, 13, 21, 307
  appearance of, 7, 22-23, 24,
    202
  barium enema x-rays with,
    222-24
  bleeding of, 193
  changes in color of, 22, 24
  changes in size of, 22, 24, 202
  of children, 208
  cleansing of, 25
  and clothing, 183
  from colostomy, 23
  from continent ostomy, 21, 299
  discharge of while cleaning,
    138
  examination of, 222
  feelings about, 61
  flush, 299
  getting used to, 50-52
  hernia around, 224, 300
  from ileostomy, 23, 91, 93,
    98, 99-100
  irregularly shaped, 123,
    126, 128, 137
  learning to manage, 8, 52-54
  locations of, 24
  measurement of, 136-37
  post-surgical behavior of,
    47-48, 51-52

  during pregnancy, 202-3,
    204
  prolapse of, 224, 306
  need for protection of, 24
  retraction of, 224, 306
  and seatbelts, 258
  during sex, 193
  surgical incision for, 74
  surgical revision of, 128,
    224. 306
  from temporary ostomy,
    150, 153-54, 160
  from urostomy, 21, 22, 23,
    48, 91, 104, 106, 107,
    111, 112
  See also Enterostomal
    therapy nurses, Mucous
    fistula, Pouches, Skin,
    Surgery
Stoma Rehabilitation Clinic, 263
Stomach, and digestion, 15
Stool, loose
  and diet, 79, 165
  and drinking water, 165
  with ileostomy, 99
  and irrigation, 76, 80
  pouches for, 117-18
  See also Diarrhea, Feces
Stool, solid, 80
  pouches for, 118
  See also Feces
Stress, 172-79
  management of, 175-79
  as natural response, 172-73
  physical consequences of,
    173-75
Stretch marks, prevention of,
  202
Supplies, ostomy
  assembling of, 135
  companies for, 116
  in developing countries,
    271, 281

Supplies, ostomy (cont.)
  expense of, 130
  and travel, 254
  See also Adhesives, Pads,
    Pouches, Skin barriers,
    Skin sealants
Support, emotional, 175
  for children, 211-12
  of family, 58, 175
  for teenagers, 217, 218, 219
  See also Emotions, Enteros-
    tomal therapy nurses,
    Openness, Support
    groups, United Ostomy
    Association
Support groups, 66, 176-77,
  199, 280-82
  and children, 211-12
  origins of, 263
  See also United Ostomy
    Association
Surgeons. See Health care
  professionals
Surgery, ostomy
  emotional recovery from, 60-66
  experience of, 7-8, 43-44, 49
  movement after, 45-46, 243
  and pain medicine, 46
  physical changes from, 50-59
  post-, 8-10, 22
  recovery from, 44-49
  See also Ostomy, Colos-
    tomy, Hospitals, Ileos-
    tomy, Pre-surgery, Uros-
    tomy
Suspenders, 182. *See also*
  Clothing
Swimming, 10, 242-43

Talking, about excretory functions, 61, 68-69
Teenagers, with ostomy, 213-19
  and autonomy, 215, 216
  and attitude, 213-14
  emotions of, 215
  and openness about os-
    tomy, 217
  and parents, 215-16
  reasons for, 214
  rejection of, 217
  special problems of, 215-16
  support for, 217, 218, 219,
    280
  with temporary ostomy, 217-18
Temporary ostomy, 15, 75,
  144-61, 307
  care of, 153-57, 159-61
  and children, 206
  difficulties of, 144
  double-barrel ostomy, 150,
    296-97
  examples of persons with,
    145-47
  loop type, 148-50; 155
  and post-surgery period, 158
  pouching techniques for,
    154-56
  reasons for, 147-48
  reconnection of, 159, 209,
    224
  stomas of, 150-51, 153-54
  surgical procedures for, 148-53
  See also Colostomy, Ileos-
    tomy, Ostomy, Undiver-
    sion, Urostomy
Tennis, 245
Tests, medical
  for cancer, 221-24
  before surgery, 33-34, 35-37
  See also Barium enema/x-
    ray, Urine tests, X-ray
Therapy. See Counseling
Thoreau, Henry David, 180
Tincture of benzoin, 52
To Build A Ship (Berry), 230
Toilet seat, and irrigation, 78-79

Toilets, portable, 257
Total Parenteral nutrition
  (TPN), 90, 98, 308
The Town Karaya, 260
Tracy, Spencer, 50
Transverse colostomy. See
  Colostomy
Travel, 250-60
  airplane, 258-60
  automobile, 258
  and camping, 256-57, 259
  and diarrhea, 255
  and diet, 255
  international, 260
  tips for, 252-57
Treatment team approach. See
  Health care professionals
Tubes, post-surgical, 46-47
Tumor boards, 229
Tumor markers, 221-22
Turnbull, Rupert, MD, 91-92,
  120, 262, 263

U.S. Department of Health
  and Human Services, 238
U.S. Federal Government
  and financial aid, 59
  and nutrition information,
    170-71
Ujhely, Gertrude, RN, 63-64
Ulcerative colitis, 5, 33, 87, 308
  and cancer risk, 89, 90, 95, 97
  causes of, 89
  in children, 206
  continent ileostomy for, 94,
    95-96, 97, 295
  and diet, 167
  ostomy as relief from, 61,
    90-91
  teenagers with, 214, 217-18
  temporary ostomies for,
    145, 146-47, 148

See also Inflammatory
  Bowel Disease
Undiversion, 103, 153, 308.
  See also Temporary Os-
  tomy
United Ostomy Association
  (UOA), 4-5, 238, 239, 270,
  273-82, 290
  and children, 211- 12
  history of, 263, 273-77
  meetings of, 183, 278
  for homosexuals/bisexuals,
    197, 280
  organization of, 277-79
  programs of, 278-81
  for singles, 197
  and teenagers, 216, 218, 219
  visitors, 27, 29-30, 38, 53,
    69, 161, 181, 271-72, 278
  See also Ostomy Quarterly
UOA. See United Ostomy
  Association
Upper GI series (x-rays), 36
Ureterostomy, 103, 152-53,
  308
Ureters, 20, 102, 103
Urethra, 20, 102; use of with
  urinary diversion, 107
Urinary diversion, 101-13, 308-9
  without stoma, 102, 107
  without stoma, in children, 207
  without stoma, temporary,
    152, 155
  See also Colonic conduit,
    Ileal conduit, Nephros-
    tomy, Ureteros tomy,
    Urostomy, Vesicostomy
Urinary tract, 309
  defects in, 20, 101, 207
  infection in, 111, 200
  reconstruction surgery for,
    103
  tests on, 36-37

Urinary Tract (cont.)
See also Bladder, Kidneys,
Ureters, Urethra, Urinary
diversion, Urine, Uros-
tomy
Urine
backflow of, 104, 106, 107,
109
crystals, 309
flow of, 104, 111, 112-13
dribbling of, 6
mucus in, 111
normal passage of, 20
pH of, 111-12
post-surgical discharge of,
47, 48.
See also Encrustation,
Incontinence, Urinary
diversion, Urinary tract,
Urostomy
Urine tests
pre-surgery, 37
regular, 111
self-administered, 112
Urologists, for sex problems,
194-95
Urostomy, 5-6, 14, 101-13, 309
and activity (physical), 247
alternatives to, 107-8
children with, 14
continent, 106-7, 217-18, 295
and drinking water, 165
management of, 108-13
need for, 20, 101-2
post-surgery experience of,
48, 108-9
and use of pouch, 108-10, 113
and pregnancy, 200
and pre-surgery medical
tests, 36-37, 108
prevalence of, 20
stoma of, 21, 22, 23, 48, 91,
104, 106, 107, 111, 112

surgical procedures for, 20-
21
temporary, 145, 147, 152-
53, 155
and travel, 251-52
See also Colonic conduit,
Ileal conduit, Night
drainage system, Tem-
porary ostomy
US Rehabilitation Act of 1973,
238

Vacuum therapy, 195-96. See
also Erection
Vesicostomy, 103, 309
Vine, Marlene, 190
Vinegar, for urine encrusta-
tion, 112.
See also Encrustation
Vinitsky, Archie, 275-76
Scholarship for ET Nursing
Education, 274
Vitamins, 163
vitamin B12, 98, 165
vitamin C, 176
Von Hugel, Freiderich, 283

Walker, Jane, ET, 98
Walking, 241, 242
and recovery from surgery,
9, 45-46
See also Exercise
Washing. See Bathing, Skin,
Stoma
Water
drinking, 99, 165
and international travel, 260
See also Dehydration, Diet,
Fluids
Weight
gain, 166
loss, 20, 87
Wells, Richard J., M.D., 61

White, Margaret, 91
Women
  special problems with sex
    of, 194
  urinary diversion for, 107
World Council of Enterostomal
  Therapy, 280

X-rays
  of digestive tract, 36, 37
  of urinary tract, 108
  See also Barium enema/x-ray

Youth Rally (United Ostomy
  Association), 218, 280

Zeit, Paul, M.D., 199, 203

Books of Related Interest

BUILDING PARTNERSHIPS IN HOSPITAL CARE: Empowering Patients, Families and Professionals, by Mary Dale Scheller, MSW. ISBN 0-923521-07-0, 324 pages, $12.95

> The author lays out a step-by-step plan for raising the quality of human caring for everyone who must spend time in hospitals and nursing homes—patients and visitors as well as health care professionals. Her unique "care partner program" draws the patient, a relative or friend, and a professional of the patient's own choosing into a mutually caring, healing partnership, to care for patients' emotional and psychological needs as well as their medical needs.

...THE DIAGNOSIS IS CANCER: A Psychological and Legal Resource Handbook for Cancer Patients, Their Families and Helping Professionals, by Edward J. Larschan, JD, PhD with Richard J. Larschan, PhD. ISBN 0-915950-77-4, 142 pages, $9.95

> "This is a guide through the twists and turns of physician selection and hospital care, legal and financial matters, and emotional roadblocks that cancer patients and their families encounter. Larschan. . . .writes with neither sentimentalism nor scare tactics, in a no-nonsense, to-the-point style. . .highly recommended for both the cancer treatment professional and layperson—to whom it is primarily directed."
>
> —*Booklist*

NUTRITION FOR THE CHEMOTHERAPY PATIENT, by Janet L. Ramstack, DrPH and Ernest H. Rosenbaum, MD. ISBN 0-915950-99-5, 420 pages, $18.95

> "This is by far the most complete and extensive book on the subject that I have seen...
>
> *Part I: Using Nutrition—How Food Can Help* is a wonderful handbook designed to empower. Filled with fact-based, information, and easy-to-read information, the tables assist in addressing very individualized patient needs, and the varied recipes take into account an array of tastes and cooking/eating styles.
>
> *Part II: Advising the Chemotherapy Patient—The Medical Prospective* is an easy-to-use reference guide for the medical practitioner. The descriptions of specific drugs assist in focusing on the unique needs of each patient."
>
> —Lyssa Friedman, RN, BSN, OCN
> Pacific Presbyterian Medical Center
> San Francisco, California

RECIPES FOR THE CHEMOTHERAPY PATIENT, by Janine Bernat, RD, Carol Stitt, RD, et. al. ISBN 0-923521-18-6, 158 pages, $12.95

> Unlike the general population, cancer patients often need to emphasize protein and calories in their diets. In addition, the side effects of drug treatments can limit tolerance to certain foods, and increase the need for foods easily swallowed and digested. These recipes were designed and tested to meet these specific needs, as well as the requirements that they be easy to plan and prepare. Originally a part of the book, *Nutrition for the Chemotherapy Patient.*